Writing, documentation and communication for nurses

Writing, documentation and communication for nurses

George Castledine

Quay
Books

Quay Books Division, Mark Allen Publishing Group, Jesses Farm, Snow Hill, Dinton, Nr Salisbury, Wiltshire, SP3 5HN
© Mark Allen Publishing Ltd, 1998

Reprinted 2003

British Library Cataloguing-in-Publication Data. A catalogue record for this book is available from the British Library

ISBN 1 85642 070 1 ✓ srb

Printed in the United Kingdom by The Cromwell Press, Wilts

Contents

Acknowledgements

Thanks to: John Peysner MA Cantab, Principal Lecturer and Solicitor, The Nottingham Trent University Law School, for his contribution to the chapter 'Legal and ethical implications'; the UKCC for permission to publish the document 'Standards for Records and Record Keeping'; and Helen Scott for editing the manuscript.

Good nursing care is your best defence against being sued for malpractice. However, if you do get into difficulties, then clear and accurate documentation of the nursing care provided will be your best defence in the courtroom.

1

Preparing to write and document

Introduction

There is no doubt that writing and documentation is one of the most important, yet most neglected, areas in nursing care. Increasingly, over the past few years, the UKCC's annual statistics have shown that poor written communication and documentation are significant factors in professional misconduct. The reasons for this are varied, but crucially it would seem that there is a general lack of advice and preparation during pre- and postregistration education. The purpose of this book, therefore, is to provide nurses with current information to help them improve their overall knowledge and skills in this area.

The book takes into consideration current factors influencing contemporary nursing charting practices. Time is a crucial issue and charting the essentials, without getting lost in unnecessary dialogue, is the key to success. Since the early days of the nursing process, some 20 years ago, nursing documentation has become increasingly important, especially in relation to legal issues.

Professional responsibility and accountability are among the most important reasons why nurses should write and document more accurately. Nurses not only are accountable to the UKCC for their actions but also have contractual accountability to their employers, as well as being accountable in law. The *Code of Professional Conduct* (UKCC, 1992a) sets out the terms of the nurse's professional accountability and to whom and how she/he is answerable. The first four clauses of the Code clearly state that the nurse should always put the interests of patients, clients and the public before any others:

As a registered nurse, midwife or health visitor, you are personally accountable for your practice and, in the exercise of your professional accountability, must:

1. *Act always in such a manner as to promote and safeguard the interests and well-being of patients and clients.*

2. *Ensure that no action or omission on your part, or within your sphere of responsibility, is detrimental to the interests, condition or safety of patients and clients.*

3. *Maintain and improve your professional knowledge and competence.*

4. *Acknowledge any limitations in your knowledge and competence and decline any duties or responsibilities unless able to perform them in a safe and skilled manner.*

These four clauses have particular relevance when considering the role of writing and nursing documentation.

The nurse should never rely solely on verbal communication; she/he should always validate what has been said or observed with written evidence. Without such information a serious omission may occur which can have consequences as referred to in Clause 2 of the Code.

Willingness to improve and acknowledge limitations are key factors in motivating and encouraging the nurse towards lifelong learning. With the advent of professional profiling, nurses are now expected to record their progress in relation to continuing education. Therefore, an overall understanding of writing and recording skills is essential for the nurse of today.

Tensions and ethical and legal problems are developing in relation to national priorities in health care. For example, the shift from long-term hospitalisation towards more acute hospitals and care in the community may result in nurses facing ethical dilemmas, or finding themselves in situations which demand careful documentation of facts. Today, nurses are more at risk from litigation than ever before. Risk, therefore, needs to be assessed.

Risk management refers to 'safety measures taken to protect the patient as well as the professional caregiver from chance of legal action', as defined by Fischbach (1991). The written risk management strategies that nurses should follow include: writing incident reports fully and clearly; recording verbal and telephone orders appropriately; the proper implementation of consent forms; and recording when patients refuse treatment or nursing care. However mundane or unusual an incident may seem, it is always advisable for the nurse to record it.

There are, of course, other reasons for writing in our professional lives. These include letters, memoranda, paperwork for meetings, reports, audit profiling, and papers for professional journals, research and nursing advancement. To write is to communicate. Writing is not just an expression of what we need to say and record; it is an expression of our feelings and concerns, and a way of describing and interpreting what has happened or is happening to our patients.

Documentation or record keeping is a method of formalising professional writing and assembling records to authenticate what we have done and the reasons behind our actions. The essentials of the nursing process form a valuable guide and framework, not only for the practice of nursing, but also for recording and evolving an essential link between the provision and evaluation of nursing care. There is a danger that, in the move towards greater interprofessional collaboration and the sharing of health care records, the nursing contribution will be much harder to identify and may well become lost to other more dominant medical health priorities.

Factors affecting documentation

Over the past few years there has been a dramatic increase in the number of codes and charters in use in daily life. One of the most significant of these was *The Patient's Charter* (Department of Health, 1991). Launched in October 1991, this was the first move to encourage greater patient/client involvement in health care. After a fairly mixed response, an expanded and updated version was circulated in 1995, introducing several national standards and giving further clarity to patients' rights and expectations (Department of Health, 1995). This resulted in many health care trusts issuing their own statements and targets for improved patient care. The overall result of these moves has been to encourage the general public to be more aware and critical of the health service that they are receiving.

The *Code of Professional Conduct* (UKCC, 1992a) was drawn up by the UKCC under the powers of the Nurses, Midwives and Health Visitors Act 1979 to give advice to registered practitioners in relation to their professional accountability. More recently, the UKCC has produced a booklet, *Guidelines for Professional Practice* (UKCC, 1996), which provides further guidance on the statements made within the Code. Significantly, paragraph 23 of this publication states:

> *To ensure that you gain the trust of your patients and clients, you should recognise them as equal partners, use language that is familiar to them and make sure they understand the information you are giving. Your records must also be clear, legible and accessible to the patient or client, as outlined in the UKCC's document 'Standards for Records and Record Keeping' and under the terms of the Data Protection Act 1984 and the Access to Health Records Act 1990. Written communication is as important as verbal communication.*

The increase in consumer awareness about the health care system has been further supplemented by a proliferation in the number of popular magazine articles and television shows about medical and nursing issues. Consumer demands for a higher quality service, therefore, have grown significantly and many patients and their relatives/friends are becoming more litigious. Overall, consumers are now expecting nurses to be more knowledgeable, competent and caring in their approach. Recognising a patient's or client's right to choose is clearly outlined in Clauses 1 and 5 of the UKCC's *Code of Professional Conduct,* and although the words 'advocacy' and 'autonomy' are not specifically used, they are taken up in *Guidelines for Professional Practice* (paragraphs 18–21). In this context advocacy is refered to as concern with promoting and protecting the interests of the patient and supporting a patient who refuses treatment/care.

One of the most significant professional functions of the registered nurse is the evaluation of the patient's response to nursing care and medical treatment. It is important, therefore, that nursing documentation clearly communicates this, in addition to the outcomes of health care interventions.

Nursing judgement

In the past, nursing documentation was process-orientated, ie. it tended to focus on the activities or tasks nurses performed on or with their patients. However, the development of standards and the increased emphasis on patient outcomes has created a need for nurses to emphasise and document the patient's progress or lack of progress. Therefore, the new direction in nursing documentation is towards nurses expressing their judgement more clearly and not just recording the nursing care they have given.

As the cost of health care continues to rise, greater attention needs to be paid to the evaluation of patient care outcomes as a way of defining the quality of health care. Clearly, defined outcomes direct how and when to evaluate the achievement of expected outcomes and provide a frame- work for documentation. Evaluation consists of both formative and summative assessments. Formative evaluation occurs during the provision of care and is an ongoing process. Summative evaluation occurs at the end of an activity, such as an admission, discharge or transfer to another area. Further discussion on formative and summative evaluation is included in *Chapter 5* under 'Methods of record keeping and progress notes'.

More recent innovations and developments in nursing documentation centre around the need to avoid duplication in order to save the nurse's time. Computerising nursing records is one solution, but unless nurses have skills in expressing themselves, computerised records will remain as poor as their written counterparts. Changes in any system should not be based on knee-jerk reactions to criticisms. Health care providers need to look critically at their systems of documentation and only introduce changes once a thorough assessment has been made of all the factors that are involved.

Collaboration in health care

The key word for future health care is 'collaboration'. Collaboration depends on clinical and interpersonal expertise and an understanding of the factors that can promote or impede efforts to develop relationships with colleagues. In North America there have been many reports of successful collaborative ventures. For example, on a macro level, the American Nurses' Association and the American Medical Association collaborated to form the National Joint Practice Commission (NJPC). The NJPC identified five criteria that were essential to the implementation of collaborative prac- tice in hospital settings: primary nursing; integrated patient records; the encouragement of nurse decision-making; the setting up of a Joint Practice Committee to look at overlaps in patient care; and a joint record review to explore and audit what was being communicated and by whom (NJPC, 1979).

Specialisation and nursing role developments

The following factors have exacerbated the confusion over specialisation in nursing and the future direction of the nurse's role:

◆ The need to respond dynamically and flexibly to economic and national health targets

◆ The pressure to reduce doctors' hours and to provide substitutes for the shortage of doctors

◆ The *ad hoc* development of specialisation in nursing

◆ Rapid and uncontrolled nursing role developments which have left nurses free to use whatever title they choose

◆ The language and cultural clash over the way that certain titles from other countries, eg. North America, have been used in the UK

◆ The confusion as to what the core terms 'generalist', 'specialist' and 'advanced' mean.

The Scope of Professional Practice (UKCC, 1992b) sets out the fundamental principles on which developments in the nurse's role should be based. There is no doubt that the nurse's level of competence is often judged on the basis of documented evidence relating to nursing decisions and nursing activities. The more nurses increase their scope of practice the more their scope of responsibility and accountability are questioned. There is a danger that some nurses will not think through the possible implications of taking on more medical and non-nursing duties. The following questions should, therefore, be carefully considered:

1. Am I knowledgeable and competent enough to be carrying out this function?

2. Is it in the best interests of the patient that I should be doing it?

3. Have I the time to do this properly and how will it affect the other essential aspects of my role?

4. How should I document my extended actions and the effect they have had on the patient?

Careful recording and written monitoring of developments in the nurse's scope of practice is important for not only the future direction of the profession but also the patient's safety. Continuity and quality of health care can be improved when nurses are flexible in their roles, but this must not be to the detriment of nursing.

The importance of a 'nursing' emphasis in documentation

It is important for the future health care of our patients that we continually strive to identify and develop nursing. One of the key problems in nursing is related to its definition. According to McFarlane and Castledine (1982):

The word 'nursing' has different derivations and meanings in different languages and in some languages there is no word for it. Although there may be a common core of function, in

7

> *different cultures the role and function of the nurse may vary*
> *widely.*

To help guide practitioners in their documentation of nursing care, the key characteristics of nursing as it is viewed in the UK must be examined. It is important that we accept, if not a simple all-embracing definition of nursing, at least several key statements about the properties that contribute to our understanding of the nature of nursing.

If we are unable to give some direction to what we mean by nursing, then what nurses write will be lost or influenced by other non-nursing decision-makers. It is critical for the patient's future quality of care that nurses write about their unique contribution. As Diers (1994) states:

> *Nursing does not defy definition; it is simply so huge that it*
> *cannot be distilled satisfactorily into one or two pithy*
> *sentences.*

In the early 19th century, nursing broadly encompassed the activities associated with maintenance of health among family members and their care in times of illness. Florence Nightingale (1859) focused the nurse's role on tasks based on the principles of hygiene, health and Christian character development. This strongly authoritarian model, practised primarily by women, led in the 1950s and 1960s to definitions of nursing centred around tasks. So important did these functions become that nurses in training in Great Britain at that time had to keep a record of proficiency in such skills and take a practical examination away from the ward area.

This functional approach continues to cause misunderstanding and confusion about the role of the nurse today. Hard-core traditionalists believed that nursing was primarily about helping patients with their basic functions and keeping strictly to current rules and principles of hygiene. The nursing theorists may have evolved as a reaction to this narrow perspective. The most notable of these theorists were Henderson, Peplau, Abdellah, Hall and Orem.

◆ Henderson (1966) suggests that nursing has a specialised role in decision-making and action related to aspects of human living. She believes that nursing focuses on the ability of the patient to fulfil the requirements of daily living and that the nurse's role is to assist the individual — sick or well — in that task. Orem, Roper, Logan and Tierney all agree that nursing is, in essence, concerned with a needs-based approach.

◆ Other nurse theorists, such as King, Orlando, Peplau and Travelbee, emphasise a more interactionist approach, placing importance on the nurse/patient relationship.

◆ A third group of nurse theorists — Roy, Johnson, Levine and Rogers — emphasise what Meleis (1985) terms the outcomes approach. They see the goal of nursing care as bringing back balance and stability, preserving energy, or enhancing harmony between the individual and her/his environment. The author has been particularly interested in this approach and has used the Roy Adaptation Model in the past (Castledine, 1986).

These three classifications of nursing theorists demonstrate the theoretical basis of present-day nursing trends but do little to help us find a simple definition of nursing. In fact, the presence of so many theories probably causes greater confusion and misunderstanding about the nature of nursing.

Properties of nursing

The following are a series of statements about the properties of nursing which may contribute to our understanding of its nature:

1. Nursing is culturally and economically determined

2. In a complex society, nursing is divided up into various specialist roles

3. As nursing becomes acceptable in a society, it develops and seeks a knowledge base which eventually becomes more exclusive and concerned with professionalisation

4. The root meaning of the word 'nurse' is nourish and a simple definition of nursing is closely related to nurturing

5. Nursing is about meeting the problems and concerns relating to bodily human functioning

6. Nursing is concerned with mental and emotional health, and spiritual problems and concerns

7. One of the major goals of nursing is to help people with their physical, emotional and mental health problems/ concerns, thus enabling them to adapt and cope with change

8. Nursing is about being present, available and perceptive to those who are having difficulties or problems in caring for themselves

9. Nursing is an interactive process emphasising an interpersonal relationship and a shared experience in health-related matters

10. Nursing has high moral and ethical standards of which accountability, autonomy, advocacy, collaboration and a duty to care are key elements

11. Nursing aims to protect the public and respect the laws of the land

12. Nursing involves educating for health, ie. aiding health promotion and disease prevention

13. Nursing is concerned with social policies and political decisions that may affect the health of those for whom we are caring

14. Nursing is an eclectic discipline, ie. it derives its ideas from various sources and is not attached to any particular school of philosophy.

Just as conceptual models can be researched, so can statements about the nature of nursing be explored. Some of these statements are new, some will change, and others will be proven to be key elements of nursing in the future. What matters is the value we place on them and our willingness to monitor and evaluate them so that they remain relevant to our nursing care.

One of the key statements above (No. 4) refers to a definition of nursing based on 'nurturing'. The word nurturing is used to denote the special caring, supporting, advocating, protecting, promoting, assisting, relieving, loving and hoping interactions that are peculiar to nursing. The list of words or terms associated with nurturing is as long as we agree to make it. Therefore, nursing documentation must reflect the values implied in the above statements, and the definition of nursing as nurturing. If nurses are not writing about these elements of care then the question must be asked: What does the nurse do?

Key principles of written communication

The ability to express oneself succinctly is a general but important skill that every nurse must possess. Verbosity, especially in patients' progress notes, may lead to difficulties in the nurse putting across her/his message. It is important to get the balance right so that intended users have sufficient information for their purposes.

Three important principles of general written communication that the writer should consider are:

1. **Who is going to use or read the information?**

   The use of professional jargon is acceptable when the intended audience is in the same profession as the writer, but in nursing care the users of nursing records may be from a much wider field. Clearly written entries help caregivers and care supporters, and the patients themselves, to see and understand what is happening. If the patient is the user, the nurse should make sure that her/his style and expressions are appropriate to that individual.

2. **What type of information does the reader require?**

   The nurse should consider what the user of the information will want to know. This may be the effects of medical treatment, technical detail, nursing care or general information about the patient and her/his progress. Nursing records are used by all members of the health care team who may not need to know every detail. Therefore, the nurse should consider the different needs of the individual people. For example, patients may not want to read all the nursing information about themselves. Clear case summaries and evaluations are often all that they want; therefore, the nurse should write these according to the patient's needs and understanding. Sometimes, writing down information in the patient's own language or dialect helps the nurse to understand the patient's culture. What has been written can usually only be judged by the way in which it is used. Lelean (1973) found that in the past nurses wrote very little information down. More recently, however, the content of nursing records has expanded and good examples of nursing documentation exist which not only have been used by nurses for professional reasons but also have been helpful in legal disputes and questions pertaining to the quality of health care.

3. **The importance of organisation and presentation of material**

It is all very well writing down accurately aspects of patient information but if they are not well organised and presented they may get lost or ignored. Planned presentation of patient information is the key to effective written and verbal reporting. Information should be appropriately organised into the relevant stages of the nursing process. This enables the user to find all information relating to certain subjects and aspects of care in one particular section. Most technical data, especially those relating to observations and medical technology, should be recorded on the relevant assessment charts. Transferring some of this information onto patients' progress notes may only be appropriate if it is significant and helps to clarify or emphasise a particular point. Without some type of agreed system or framework for charting different aspects of patient care, the nurse may experience confusion and frustration with regard to her/his record keeping.

It may be helpful for the nurse to consider presenting data in terms of categories. For example:

(i) Time, eg. chronological sequence of events or time of occurrence

(ii) Problems, eg. nursing problems, medical problems, patient-perceived problems, social problems

(iii) Stages, eg. critical, acute, rehabilitation, chronic

(iv) Dependency, eg. totally or partially dependent on nurse, self-caring or independent.

Whatever system is used the important point is the need to organise and present data so that they can be found easily and read without difficulty.

Using plain words

Sir Ernest Gowers (1956), in his classic work on the importance of using plain words, stated:

> *The basic fault of present-day writing is a tendency to say what one has to say in as complicated a way as possible. Instead of being simple, terse and direct, it is stilted, longwinded, and circumlocutory; instead of choosing the simple word it prefers the unusual, instead of the plain phrase the cliché.*

Nurses are as guilty of this as any other group of professional people in society today. They certainly need to reduce the amount of 'jargon' in their writing. Several pressure groups now exist who are concerned with the way we use or abuse our native languages, eg. the Plain English Society and the Welsh Language Society. Official forms, public information sheets, commercial documents, insurance policies and health care information are all coming under closer scrutiny. There are many cultural and language differences throughout the UK and therefore nurses must be more careful and effective when dealing with different ethnic groups. In order to avoid cultural-based errors in communication nurses must accept all human beings for who they are and remember that health beliefs and health behaviours are often culturally defined.

It is important to follow and assess the patient's individual behaviour carefully. Writing down key health care words and their translation is helpful not only for the patient but also for the nurse. The use of jargon, colloquialism and slang should be avoided.

The general rule of using short words that everybody understands (see *Figure 1.1*) is helpful when dealing with different cultural groups. Short sentences are better than long ones. Writing and documenting well takes time. Often nurses become impatient, try to avoid the task, copy others or use well-worn, subjective and meaningless phrases.

Figure 1.1: Examples of short words	
Do not put:	**If you could put:**
purchase	buy
inculate	teach
commence	start
extraordinary	odd
magnitude	size
quantify	measure
transmit	send
immediately	now
proceed	go on
utlise	use
categories	kinds
reimburse	repay
activate	start
eradicate	erase
implement	carry out
initiate	begin
maximum	most
minimum	least
optimum	best
terminate	end, conclude
validate	prove

As the emphasis is now on reflective practice it is much more acceptable for nurses to admit their limitations and to try to improve themselves. Nurses should ask a mentor to check carefully what they have written and give them feedback. It is also useful to examine other people's style of writing. The importance of correct spelling cannot be overemphasised.

Figure 1.2: Translating abstractions and verbosities

It is better to replaceabstract nouns with verbs, concrete nouns or other words. The way to recognise the worst abstract noun is by examining their endings: -ion; -tion; -ility; -nce; -ment; -ship; -itude.

Do not write:	If you could write
give consideration to	consider
on a regular basis	regularly
a substantial part	much
are not in a position to	cannot
is a clear vindication of	justifies
transportation facilities	porters or messengers
providing information	informing
entrance location	door
in the eventuality of	if
on the assumption that	if
communications	messages, memos, letters
given instruction	teach, tell, describe
poor mobility	difficulty walking
skin integrity impaired	poor skin condition
home maintenance management impaired	unable to do housework
breathing pattern difficulty	breathing problems
sexual dysfunction	impotent
social interaction impairment	deaf, dumb, blind
poor attitude to comradeship	likes living alone
health-seeking behaviour	wants to know
knowledge deficit	not to be informed
the human factor	people

As it is important to write plainly and clearly, *Figure 1.2* lists words that can be used as alternatives to more abstract nouns. No-one can write good English just by knowing the rules of grammar and syntax. The most important factor is the individual writer's choice of words. Therefore, it is up to nurses to decide for themselves which word best expresses a nursing or patient care situation. In some cases, however, it is more appropriate for the nurse to use a direct quotation from the patient, especially when writing patient responses in the progress notes (see *Chapter 5*).

Punctuation

Whole books have been written on the subject of punctuation. It would seem that no two authorities completely agree on its usage. The following is a brief guide.

Nurses generally underpunctuate. In writing reports and recording notes, nurses are frequently encouraged to use incomplete sentences and short descriptive statements.

As Gower (1956) points out:

Taste and common sense are more important than any rules; you put in stops to help your reader to understand you, not to please grammarians.

As long as the nurse uses full stops, commas and quotation marks appropriately, then this should be sufficient to convey the correct meaning. For example, full stops should be used to divide up sentences which need to be kept short and simple to convey meaning. The main uses of the comma are:

1. Between adjectives, eg. a cautious, eloquent person

2. To separate items in a list

3. To mark the beginning and end of a phrase

Quotation marks are very important in the recording and reporting of patient and client information. The use of single or double quotation marks is considered a matter of personal preference or house style. Quotation marks express what someone else has said or written and demonstrate patient involvement, ie. what the patient really is saying and thinking. They must always be used when introducing direct speech, eg. The patient said, 'I have a burning pain'. Punctuation, when used well, will certainly enhance the nurse's written communication skills. This information is intended only as a guide to some of the essentials.

Non-sexist writing

Sometimes the way in which language is used offends people. It is important that nurses are sensitive to this in their documentation. There is no place for sexism in nursing and health care, and it is important for all health care team members to get into the habit of thinking carefully about when to use masculine and feminine terms. Today, many organisations have a policy of non-sexist writing and some businesses and local authorities apply the policy compulsorily. In health and nursing situations the patient is often referred to as 'he', the nurse as 'she', and the doctor as 'he'. In nursing, to refer to a man as a 'male nurse' may be offensive to some people, depending upon the situation and the circumstances in which it is used.

A rough guideline of what is acceptable is whether the practice would be right if reversed. Thus, it may sound strange to say, 'she is a female nurse'. Therefore, we should not use 'she' for a person who might be a man or a boy. Neither should we use masculine terms such as 'he' when the person might be a woman or girl, or 'man' to mean 'men or women'. Masculine pronouns such as 'him' and 'his' should only be used in a masculine, not a universal, sense. Examples of non-sexist writing are illustrated in *Figure 1.3*.

Figure 1.3: Examples of non-sexist writing	
Do not write:	**Do write:**
Dear Miss/Mrs	Dear Ms or begin a letter with Dear Florence Nightingale. Dear John Smith is also acceptable when writing to a man and more personal than Dear Sir of Mr.
man-hours	working hours or staff hours
manpower	workers, labour force, staff
Dear Chairman	If not a man or not sure write Dear Chair or Chairperson
you and your husband	you and your partner

As language is changing continually we are probably in a state of transition on this subject. Therefore, a full set of non-sexist alternatives may not be available yet. The following, however, are some suggested alternatives:

From: A nurse feels that she should have equal rights.

To: A nurse feels that he or she should have equal rights.

Or: Nurses feel that they should have equal rights.

Or: A nurse may want equal rights.

In other words, go for the longer version 'he or she' or 'him or her', the plural 'they', or reword the sentence. All this may seem a little over-cautious but it is important to be sensitive to other people's preferences and avoid the risk of offending the feelings and ideals of your reader.

Summary

Many changes are taking place in nursing and the health care environment. Such events or trends will continue to place a burden on documentation and communication in nursing. Nurses, therefore, need to keep up to date and remain flexible, dynamic and responsive to change. Documentation outcomes and policies should always reflect the reality of what is happening in practice. The nursing contribution to care must be identified and emphasised in all aspects of written communication and record keeping. It is important that nurses follow a particular system and record the essential aspects of nursing assessment, problem identification, planning and patient evaluation. Writing or typing concisely and precisely takes time, but if nurses follow the key points and essential factors they will quickly develop their knowledge and competency.

This text has been designed to outline the principles on which good documentation standards can be developed. The importance of nursing judgement is emphasised, as is the autonomy of the nurse and patient. Essential points are grouped together for quick reference and convenience.

The UKCC acknowledges that nurses should be more aware of the importance of their records and communication skills. There is still an alarming number of nurses getting into trouble because of their poor documentation and written communications. Therefore, information from the UKCC is included in this text (see *Chapter 4*).

No one particular documentation system is proposed, only the underlying principles that maintain and improve standards and thus preserve individuality and creativity in practice.

2

Communication skills and documentation

Human communication, key concepts and stages

Human communication is about trying to establish contact, meaning and an exchange of information. The process is a complex one and many factors are involved.

Nurses must realise that although we are principally a verbal society, we are also a literate one. Written information is crucial in our lives for the recording of aspirations, feelings and facts. The expression of this link between our thoughts and utterances and documentation, although easy for some, often needs developing in others, particularly when the individual is too weak, handicapped, or sick to record her/his own health care history and nursing needs. It is the nurse's primary responsibility to communicate with patients and to liaise and advocate for them. This involves establishing a meaningful relationship which will facilitate the patient's relevant past and present health and nursing history. The accurate recording of this information, and subsequent additions, is made easier when the nurse has mastered some of the key communication skills outlined in this chapter.

One of the most common problems for nurses is their failure to assign the right meaning to a message received from a patient. For example, imagine a typical ward scene in which a nurse is caring for several postoperative patients. The nurse is keen to finish all the observations so that she can start something else, and therefore conveys a hurried and harassed attitude to one of the patients who is in severe discomfort. She glances across at the patient and asks him if he is okay. He nods his head slightly while biting his lower lip. The nurse interprets this as non-complaining and records a satisfactory postoperative progress in the patient's notes.

The emphasis on good communication skills as the basis for good nursing care has always been a feature of nursing. Florence Nightingale said:

Always sit down when a sick person is talking business to you. Show no signs of hurry, give complete and full consideration if your advice is wanted and go away the moment the subject is ended. Always sit within the patient's view... Never speak to an invalid from behind, or from the door, or from any distance from him nor when he is doing something (Nightingale, 1859).

The key concepts to consider are:

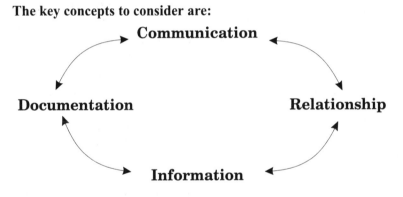

Although it is true that many nurses are naturally good at getting on with people it does not follow that they will all be good communicators. Natural ability plays a part, but everyone can learn from reviewing the ground rules and from an appraisal of their communication skills. A common misconception is that pressure of time and inadequate clinical facilities are the reasons why nurses do not communicate well with their patients/clients. These factors may hamper communication but they are insufficent reasons for not trying to improve communication skills.

Initial stage

Effective communication begins with establishing a rapport with the patient. This is often referred to as the beginning or orientation stage in the nurse/patient relationship. During this stage the nurse is starting to assess the patient, and the patient is exploring possibilities with the nurse. The patient needs to feel that the nurse can be trusted and that there is no pressure to divulge more information than is necessary. At this stage, the patient will probably only recount primary facts. Therefore, the nurse should follow a simple nursing history guide to elicit the main details. It is quite permissible at this stage to show the patient the nursing history record and to explain what is being recorded and why.

The nurse should encourage the patient to speak freely and not restrict her/his questions to the type that require rapid factual responses. The occasional open-ended question, which invites the patient to say what is on her/his mind, may help to demonstrate that the nurse is willing to listen. The nurse should try to see the patient's health problems from the patient's point of view. At this stage it is better to record patient information immediately, either directly on to the nursing record system or on to a pad for transfer to the system as soon as possible after the event. If writing brief notes during the interview, it is advisable to record carefully the 'key' expressive words that the patient has used.

When interviewing a patient or her/his significant others it is best to try to provide for privacy, physical comfort and freedom from interruptions. The nurse should always be sensitive to the patient's situation, observing for both verbal and non-verbal expressions, changes in mood and difficulties in answering any of the questions. There is often a tendency, particularly marked in doctors, to use technical and professional jargon when asking patients questions. The nurse must not copy this approach and should ask her/his questions in a concrete and simple way. It is important not to delve too deeply into complex issues during the first interview. The issue of confidentiality should also be discussed, and the patient told what the information will be used for and who will have access to it.

Towards the end of the first 'scene-setting' interview, the nurse should be starting to feel that the patient has confidence in her/him and that a basis is being established for a more in-depth working relationship.

Secondary stages

The next phase in the nurse/patient relationship is often referred to as the middle or working stage. It is important to stress that as this is a time of getting to know the patient, this phase should stretch over the period that the nurse is in direct contact with the patient. In some situations it may be appropriate to arrange a formal interview or progress session with the patient. However, as the nurse is often in a key position to observe the patient each day, she/he will be able to choose the most appropriate time to talk with the patient.

During this phase patients will start to discuss their problems and feelings in more depth. Affective material will dominate and therefore the nurse needs to know how to record such information. One important tip is to pay attention to the frequency of affective words used and the way the patient behaves when offering information. Again, it is better not to sit and write verbatim notes but to write down the key affective words and, when the session is over, write up an account in the progress notes (see *Chapter 5*). Patients should be encouraged to express and analyse their feelings regarding their health concerns. The nurse should try to be as facilitative as possible, encouraging patients to identify interventions which may help them. If patients are hesitant or reluctant to discuss their concerns, then the nurse should encourage them to write down their questions and worries so that they can be expressed at a later stage with an appropriate nurse or member of the health care team.

Many patients are alarmed by consultants' ward rounds and it is the nurse's role, both during and after these, to support and encourage patients to express their concerns.

Nurses working on night duty should be particularly sensitive to patients' needs and record carefully in the progress records specific anxieties the patient may have, particularly in relation to sleep. Very little has been written on the importance of night nurses' written records. However, their contribution is essential if we are to gain a complete picture of the patient's progress. Specific reference should be made in a patient's care plan to nursing interventions carried out during the night. In addition, relevant incidents that have occurred during this time should be described. Often, nurses only record their opinions of how well patients have slept. It is important to demonstrate that the patient has been consulted and therefore it is advisable to quote directly what the patient feels about her/his sleep and rest.

Nurses need to learn how to reassure and maintain hope in patients. The essence is to concentrate on the positive aspects of recovery or past helpful ways of coping. If patients do not feel that they are making progress, then their progress as charted in their records can be fed back to them.

When patients are talking freely and relevantly about their concerns, the nurse is achieving several important goals. First, she/he is enabling them to ventilate their true feelings, which may be all that patients need in order to feel that they are in control of their own situation. Second, by airing any problems, both nurse and patient gain a clearer picture of the situation. Third, the nurse is able to record notes that are pertinent to the patient's true feelings. Finally, the patient is enabled to verbalise her/his feelings and, by reading the nurse's notes, reflect on her/his problems.

It is during this secondary stage in the nurse/patient relationship that the nurse is able to help clients begin to understand the nature of their problems and the ways in which they can find appropriate solutions.

The recording of key patient problems and relevant actions and goals is not only good professional nursing, but also a way of enabling the patient and relevant others to review what is happening. In the case of an unconscious patient, the nurse should encourage relevant family and friends to be involved in the decision-making process. Helping patients to make key decisions about their health care is an important goal of nursing. Writing down the extent to which the patient or family has been involved in the care process is an excellent way of evaluating the quality of patient self-determination and autonomy.

Final stage

The final stage in the nurse/patient relationship is critical but is often the least emphasised. This stage is sometimes referred to as the 'terminator' or the resolution phase. Patients often complain that they are interviewed and assessed by a nurse at the start of their hospitalisation but that this does not occur at the end. It is sometimes difficult for nurses to draw a relationship with a patient to a close. To help facilitate this, certain strategies can be used. The nurse can summarise and, with the help of the patient's written record, evaluate how effective the nursing care and health promotion strategies have been in relation to recovery. It may also be helpful to write a summary of the patient's progress and nursing care, not only on the relevant discharge documents but also in the patient's records. A clear and accurate summary reinforces the effect of the progress made and enhances the sense of improvement, which is important for not only patients and their family and friends but also the nursing staff and other members of the health care team.

The nurse should help the patient to tolerate the discomfort associated with breaking away from the patient/nurse relationship and the security which a hospital can bring. Involving patients in a reflective, written review of their health care progress will enable them to make a more positive transition to the next stage of their care.

Factors for good therapeutic relationships with patients

Non-verbal variables which affect both the patient and the nurse include the use of eye contact, facial expression, posture, bodily movements, touch, appearance, dress, pitch, rate and volume of voice, gestures and distance and positioning when preparing to speak. A slouched posture can suggest lack of energy or interest, as can failure to look at the person directly. It is also important to consider patients' social background, education and culture as these may affect the way in which they communicate and interact.

The primary variables that affect the communication process are perception, self-esteem and attending behaviours.

Perception is a complex process by which all of us select, organise and interpret sensory stimuli in a meaningful way (Sereno and Bodakin, 1975). Therefore, when a nurse organises information into meaningful parts and edits it, she/he does so in the context of her/his past experiences, attitudes and values.

Self-esteem is the key to an individual's sense of worth. During interactions with other people we are often confirming or affirming their individual view of themselves.

Attending behaviours are those activities which help the nurse focus on the patient and which encourage effective, two-way communication. Examples are eye contact, body position and use of encouragement through non-verbal cues.

Empathy is understanding another person's situation or feelings. Egan (1976) describes the good communicator as an active participant who is perceptive to verbal and non-verbal cues, who clarifies what is sensed and who builds on that information to develop understanding.

Key empathic skills

- ◆ Listening to the patient
- ◆ Encouraging the patient to talk
- ◆ Using silence and attention to encourage responses from patients
- ◆ Not being condescending or patronising in manner or verbal response
- ◆ Being objective and open, not judgemental
- ◆ Not giving unsolicited advice
- ◆ Not using professional jargon and clichés
- ◆ Encouraging respect by asking relevant and key questions

◆ Encouraging a shared balance of control and power by letting the patient feel important by making a worthwhile contribution.

Source: Egan (1976).

Apart from these suggestions, it is also important to convey reciprocal trust and to make a sincere effort to understand how patients view their world and their experiences, and the meaning they attach to them. The following acronym high-lights key pointers for encouraging patients to express their feelings:

Soler

S   — *face the person Squarely*

O   — *adopt an Open posture*

L   — *Lean towards the person*

E   — *maintain good Eye contact*

R   — *be at home and relatively Relaxed in this position.*

Helpful and hindering communication techniques

Helpful techniques

◆ Use open-ended question, ie. questions that present the patient with options for response other than 'yes' or 'no'

◆ Avoid closed questions, ie. when the answer is implied in the question

◆ Reflect back to patients what they have said as this can help direct and clarify significant or confusing remarks

◆ After communicating empathy to the patient help the patient identify and explore alternatives

◆ Share observations as this can be helpful for patients. say things like 'You appear rather sad?' as this can help the patient at the start of an interview

- ◆ Encourage the patient to continue speaking by using verbal cues such as 'Go on' or 'You were saying', or non-verbal cues such as nodding and raising your eyebrows
- ◆ Give the patient feedback and summarise what you think she/he has been talking about.

Hindering techniques

- ◆ Using paternalistic and judgemental words
- ◆ Using terms the patient does not understand
- ◆ Trying to indoctrinate the patient
- ◆ Failing to clarify adequately something in the conversation which seems key to the patient
- ◆ Trying to take control of the situation
- ◆ Writing all the time and not looking at the patient
- ◆ Failing to focus on the patient's concerns
- ◆ Giving ineffective or inappropriate reassurance
- ◆ Not providing an explanation for the reasons why information has been solicited as this may lead to a breakdown in communication
- ◆ Not keeping to the subject, switching the topic or conversing at a superficial level
- ◆ Appearing to be rushed or hurried with too little time to speak with the patient.

Taking notes during nurse/patient interactions

Some nurses write nothing during their interviews and discussions with patients but make more detailed notes immediately afterwards. It is unwise to delay as you run the risk of forgetting important points that arose early in the conversation. There is no perfect solution to this problem but on balance you should be prepared to take notes and you should ask the patient in advance whether she/he minds. With experience you will find that you can record sufficient information while the patient is talking without interrupting the flow. You will develop your own form of shorthand. There are times, however, when you should not take notes. If your manner has encouraged the patient to confide personal matters, which are clearly important or distressing, you should put down your pen. If you want to make a note of this do so later when the patient is talking about something less important or immediately after the interview.

From time to time you may find yourself in conversation with an exceedingly talkative patient who finds it difficult to focus on her/his real problems. There is no easy or straightforward solution to this problem and you will have to use your own judgement when trying to redirect the course of the conversation. There is no doubt that you will have to interrupt, but not in the middle of a sentence; wait for a suitable moment and then say, 'Thank you, that was very interesting. I wonder if you could now just give me a summary of what happened after that; I'd like to get the overall picture first and then we can come back to just those particular points'. Other useful phrases include, 'Fine, so that brings us up-to-date, can I now ask you to tell me... ' or 'Could we now turn to... ' or, in extreme cases, 'Can I now ask you to jump ahead to... '. Do not forget to round off and close conversations and interviews with patients and to inform them, if necessary, of the purpose of your written notes.

All forms of communications about patients and their care must be truthful and within the bounds of confidentiality. It is important for the nurse to remember that all patient information is confidential. Nursing records are only for the eyes of nurses, their employers and certain members of the health care team. Any oral conversations about the patient should be restricted to the appropriate places and circumstances, eg. the change of shift report.

Using professional jargon

The dictionary definition of jargon is: 'Unintelligible words, gibberish; barbarous or debased language...speech familiar only to a group or profession'.

As nursing develops its scientific base and modern medical technology progresses, so the need to explain discoveries, ideas and developments increases. This often means that those who make these discoveries and the professionals who use them modify and invent new words to describe and explain the ideas. Gowers (1956), in his classic work *The Complete Plain Words,* states:

Really there are times when I feel that civilisation will come to an end because no-one will understand what anybody else is saying.

Using jargon is a dangerous habit as it interferes with communication. However, nurses can easily slip into using it when either writing or talking to patients and non-nurses. There is no doubt that nursing is developing and refining its own professional terminology and that it is being heavily influenced by the languages of medicine, educational theory and the social sciences. When parts of a professional vocabulary become pretentious and unnecessarily complex or obscure, they no longer serve a useful purpose. At this point the language passes from the realm of acceptable professional terminology into jargon.

A possible reason why some nurses use jargon is because they want to sound professional. Sometimes people use jargon when they do not really know what it means. Jargon becomes a defence, used by writers as a front to sound important and knowledgeable.

Examples of abbreviations used by nurses

- ◆ Cath for catheterisation
- ◆ Staph for staphylococcus infection
- ◆ Pre-op for preoperation
- ◆ Post-op for postoperation
- ◆ IV for an intravenous infusion
- ◆ PR for per rectum
- ◆ PV for per vagina
- ◆ Lap for laparotomy

◆ MI for myocardial infarction.

It is important that nurses stop and ask themselves, 'Am I falling into the jargon trap without realising it?'

The easiest way to avoid jargon is to express ideas simply and forcefully. The key is to be clear, concise and accurate, checking that the language used will be understood by those for whom it is intended. Professional language must be simple and direct.

Documentation and reporting

The process and the quality of exchanging information between members of the health care team, and others, has long been a source of concern. Lelean (1973) found that ward reports tended to be a one-way process (from sister to the nurses), and stated that nurses should be taught to think of each patient's care in total and not just as a series of tasks to be performed:

Hospitals should consider developing a policy for reports, both written and verbal, and all members of staff need to receive adequate training in their function and use.

Just how far we have developed our record keeping over the past 20 years or so is debatable.

Reports offer a summary of activities or observations that have been seen, performed or heard. There are five types of report made by nurses. These are:

1. Handover reports.

2. Audit reports.

3. Telephone reports.

4. Discharge/transfer reports.

5. Incident reports.

The basic routine for writing reports should be the collection of information, analysing it and then reporting it to others (Fletcher and Gowing, 1987).

1. Handover reports

The number and type of handovers are dependent on the location of the nursing care being provided. In hospital, handover may occur two or three times a day, whereas in the community it may occur only when the practitioner is going on holiday or study leave. There are a variety of methods which can be used when carrying out a handover. As mentioned earlier, Lelean (1973) found that handover was predominantly an oral, one-way process, with recipients writing down notes in pocket books for later reference.

Following the introduction of the nursing process and primary nursing, the patient's named nurse or shift nurse is the person who usually gives the report, either at the patient's bedside or in the ward conference room. The nurse should review systematically the patient's problems, nursing interventions and relevant details. It is important that the ward coordinator (eg. the ward sister) directs and chairs these sessions. Reports given in this way enable the rest of the nursing team to ask questions. Bedside reports give the patient and family members the opportunity to participate in, and contribute to decisions. Any sensitive information which may alarm the patient should be reported out of hearing.

In the community, as well as in some hospital situations, the patient keeps her/his own records, and ongoing information is completed collaboratively. Time restrictions for handovers mean that information has to be passed on quickly and efficiently. The following are some key points:

1. Always refer to the written records and use them in your presentation.

2. Organise records so that they are easy to follow.

3. If the people you are presenting to know the patient, do not spend time reviewing the biographical details.

4. Identify the patient's main nursing problems and the related causes.

5. Describe objective measurements, observations or evidence about the patient's condition and response.

6. Stress recent changes.

7. Draw attention to any particular written directives, patient requests, or allergic responses.
8. Do not review all routine care.
9. Ensure that new staff are briefed fully on the patient's problems and care needs.
10. Do not engage in idle gossip and wander from the point of the report.
11. Finally, it is important when handover sessions are carried out that all members of the team respect confidentiality and avoid labelling patients and family members as uncooperative, difficult, manipulative or awkward.

Patient care conferences are another method of conducting a handover report is to hold a patient care conference. This may include a variety of health care team members, the patient/client and her/his family/friends. This type of conference is an ideal opportunity for passing on information about a patient when transferring or discharging a case. It can also be used as a vehicle for evaluation, audit and nurse clinical supervision.

2. Audit reports

Every health care institution or trust should regularly review information in patient and client records in order to evaluate the quality and appropriateness of the care provided. In nursing terms it is important that the standards set by the UKCC are followed (see *Chapter 4*). A simple audit tool can be used (see *Chapter 4*). Nurses should monitor or review records throughout the year to determine the degree to which quality assurance and quality improvement standards have been met. Any deficiencies during this process should be shared with all members of the nursing staff so that corrections in policy or practice can be made. Where multidisciplinary records or collaborative care planning are being used it is important that the nursing contribution is audited and evaluated.

When compiling an audit report the nurse should follow a particular structure in her/his written presentation:

- Introduction to the subject, with reference to audit work and its purpose
- An outline (under headings) of the main findings and conclusions
- Key weaknesses or problems found
- Circumstances and possible reasons for problems found
- Present policy and relationship to local and national standards
- Recommendations and an assessment of the costs and savings of methods or measures to improve the situation
- Pictures, graphs, diagrams, etc. can be very helpful. A good report will only succeed as a piece of effective writing if the writer has a clear understanding of the needs of those who are going to read it. So make sure it is relevant, precise and concise.

3. Telephone reports

A nurse should be careful when giving or receiving information over the telephone, in particular verbal orders. It is important that a permanent record is made of what has been said and, in the case of patient information, a note made of the patient's details such as name, address, unit number, diagnosis and any relevant distinguishing features. Unclear sentences or information should be repeated back; this is particularly important when receiving prescription details. Depending on the nature of the information being imparted, ask a colleague to listen to a repeat of it. Documentation should occur during and immediately after the call, noting the date and time of the call and the names of those involved.

The giving of advice to a patient over the telephone should also be carefully recorded. Clearly determine the patient's/client's name. If the person seems hurried or anxious it is advisable to ask questions that clarify the situation so that no misunderstandings occur. If the patient appears to be experiencing a serious medical or nursing problem, she/he should be instructed to attend the emergency department as soon as possible.

4. Discharge/transfer reports

Transferring a patient/client from one health care facility to another is often referred to as 'discharge'. This is an unfortunate term as it suggests that the nurse has completed all the nursing care required and that the case is finished. In many situations this is not the case; it is therefore important to pass on vital patient information so that nursing care can continue uninterrupted. The completion of a special transfer summary report is one of the best ways of ensuring that information is passed on. Nurses on the receiving end of a transfer report need the following information:

♦ A brief summary of the patient and her/his nursing and medical problems/concerns

♦ The most current information about the patient's/ client's progress

♦ Any relevant and successful care plans, nursing interventions or special equipment used

♦ Any critical assessments or interventions to be completed shortly after transfer. This helps the receiving nurse to maintain continuity of care and establish priorities.

5. Incident reports

Regardless of which term a health care agency, trust or an institution may choose, an incident is defined as, 'any event that is not consistent with the usual operation of the agency or with the routine care of the patient' (Fischbach, 1991). It is a circumstance that has the potential to cause, or actually has caused, damage to people and/or property. Such incidents are usually related to errors, environmental hazards, or equipment malfunctions.

Falls are among the most frequent accidents that occur in health care delivery settings, eg. from beds, out of wheelchairs, in bathrooms and corridors, on wet floors, against doors or furniture, or over obstacles on the floor.

In the past, incident reporting — or, more specifically, filling out an incident report — was viewed as a negative activity. This may still be the case today. However, incident reporting has positive and beneficial functions. An incident report helps to identify risk in order to improve patient care and makes it possible to investigate and correct potential areas of liability so that similar instances do not happen again. As an educational aid it can help in certain kinds of client/ patient teaching and nursing care. The evaluation of incident reports provides useful information for instituting not only preventative measures but also training needs.

An error in a patient's medication treatment or nursing care also requires the nurse to submit an incident report. Currently, any mishap involving a patient should be considered very carefully and a report filled in, even if there is no apparent injury. This is also the case for incidents involving visitors and employees.

When an incident occurs, the nurse involved in the incident or the nurse who witnessed it should first take steps to remove the individual from further risk, without putting her/himself at risk. A physician must then be called to determine whether any injury has been suffered; this examination should be recorded in the client's medical record. An incident form should then be filled in by the nurse involved in the incident or the nurse who witnessed it. The witnessing nurse should only document an objective description of what she/he actually saw and any follow-up care that occurred. Some health care agencies have one form for patients, employees and visitors, whereas others use separate forms for visitors and employees.

An incident report should be concise and accurate, reporting exactly what the nurse observed and administered in the way of nursing care and aid. Regardless of what format an incident report takes, there are key guidelines to follow:

1. The nurse who witnessed the event or who found the client at the time of the incident should record:

   i) The type of incident, eg. fall, accidentally striking oneself with a needle, equipment malfunction, etc.

   ii) Detail about the people involved

   iii) Time of discovery

   iv) Place of discovery

   v) Witness(es)

vi) Observations of patient, visitor, employee and/or environment

vii) A description of what she/he saw, in concise and objective terms

viii) The patient's/client's condition when the incident was discovered

ix) Any measures taken and who the incident was reported to, including notifying the physician and her/his subsequent visit

x) Précis of the care given to the client after the incident.

2. The nurse should not interpret or attempt to explain the cause of the incident

3. Nobody should be blamed in an incident report

4. The report should be submitted as soon as possible to the appropriate senior manager.

Objective and timely reporting and recording of incidents is a valuable activity as it encourages the investigation and resolution of risks and the problems that occur as a result of these risks (Fischbach, 1991). The incident report is an internal device for the health care agency. It is considered necessary for internal use in the quality assurance programme and risk management survey.

Writing business letters

The popular image of nurses helping injured soldiers write letters home to their loved ones during the war years has long passed. Today, letter writing is usually restricted to answering complaints, appealing for funds, answering enquiries and thank yous.

Success at business writing does not come easily and requires careful thought. To ensure success, letters need to be planned, eg. deciding what needs to be said and how to say it. Letters should be personal and sincere. Business letters must be brief and to the point.

In Dickens' time business letters were crafted in long-winded and complicated language, but modern letters are much simpler.

When planning your letter think about what you want to say, identifying the main points and the supporting points. If you are responding to a letter have that letter in front of you as you write to make sure you address all the issues raised.

The appearance of a business letter, ie. the paper it is written on, the design of the letterhead and the type of writing or layout of the typing, is important as it conveys vital messages to its recipient. The quality of your trust or health care agency is transmitted in more than just the words you use.

It is essential that you keep your letter personal; remember that it is a communication between two people. Try to be as helpful as you can and use 'I' or 'we' and 'our policy ' instead of 'this writer' or 'this trust' or 'the hospital's policy'. Keep the language simple and use familiar words. Most of your sentences should be under 20 words in length. 'One idea, one sentence' is a good rule. Take a stand on what you are reporting and do not be timid. Positive statements are better than negative ones. Avoid sweeping certainties such as, 'I'm sure you understand' and words of surprise such as, 'I'm surprised you were told that'.

Never begin a letter with unpleasant news. The reader is likely to read no further or, even if she/he does, is likely to find fault with much of what you have said.

Letters of complaints

When answering complaints the general rules are — assuming that the complaint is justified — be courteous, apologise, make amends and do not upset the complainant. The challenge is to turn the situation around so that you win over a previously aggrieved individual with the quality of your response.

Letters of condolences

Keep condolences brief and send an appropriate card. If you are writing to a relative following a bereavement it is advisable to keep the letter short. Offer consolation and support.

Litigious letters

Today, nurses may find themselves in correspondence with people who are ready to sue, or at least threatening to sue. In such cases it is advisable to get legal advice but, if you do reply, you are strongly advised to head your letter **'Without prejudice'** which means that what you have said in the letter does not represent a final or unqualified statement on your part. Such a heading acts in the same way as heading a letter 'Subject to contract' when you are buying a house so that it does not represent an irrevocable offer or acceptance of an offer.

Thank you letters

Nurses often receive thank you letters but may overlook the need to send them to others for services rendered or other kindnesses. When writing such a letter remember that as a nurse you need to project an image of professionalism at all times, not only in the way you speak but also in your written communication.

Key points relating to letters

◆ Simple letter of request:	– Facts
	– Action
◆ Simple answer of request:	– Thanks
	– Responses
◆ Complex request:	– Facts:
	Who you are
	What problem has arisen
	Possible solutions
	Reasons against certain solutions
	The best solution
	– Action:
	X to do this
	Y to do that

◆ Complex answer to request:
- Thanks
- Sympathise with the problem
- Restate important facts
- Indicate difficulties with proposed solution
- Suggest another course of action
- Indicate willingness to discuss further

◆ Letter of complaint:
- Facts:

  What happened, where, whenand theconsequences
- Action:

  What you suggest should be done

◆ Rejecting a complaint:
- Thanks for letter
- Sympathise with problem
- Agree where possible
- Disagree or question where necessary
- State rejection
- Explain in more detail
- Suggest an action

◆ Accepting a complaint:
- Thanks
- Brief apology
- Agree facts in outline
- Disagree where necessary
- What action will be taken to prevent recurrence
- Restore confidence and goodwill

Starting a letter

This section is mainly about conventions — things that exist as much for politeness as for efficiency, eg. letters starting with 'Dear...' These conventions have changed a great deal over the years and are still on the move. After 'Dear' put the name of the person to whom you are writing, taking the trouble to spell it properly. Avoid 'Dear Sir' or 'Dear Madam'. People usually like being recognised by name. You need not fear that your letter will be unanswered if the named person is away; unless you write 'Personal' on the envelope, someone at the workplace will deal with it.

Use the correct *title,* such as Mr, Mrs or Dr. Look for a title on any letter you are answering and for letters after the name (eg. address people with PhDs as 'Dr'). When writing to members of the armed services, refer to their service title, eg. Colonel. There may be special titles such as Dr or Capt. Abbreviations which exclude the last letters usually end with a full stop, eg. Rev. and Prof. Contractions which omit the middle of the word but include the last letter, do not need a full stop, eg. Mr and Dr.

Women, unless they have a special title, are Miss, Mrs, Ms. Try to find out which they prefer. If that is not possible leave the title out. If there is a first name you can write 'Dear Claire Lippett' and 'Claire Lippett, 7 Acacia Avenue' on the envelope. If you know you are writing to a woman, but there is no first name, use 'Ms' or write 'Dear Madam'. Few would write 'Dear Lippett' or 'Dear C Lippett'.

After 'Dear Name' put a *heading*. A heading helps the reader to focus on the subject of the letter, and helps others to file the letter and retrieve it. Headings should be short, usually not more than half a line. Do not use 're' in a heading (or anywhere else). You can put reference numbers such as invoice numbers or order numbers in the heading if they are helpful.

In the *first sentence* try to:

◆ Thank the person for her/his letter, or otherwise refer to some common experience, knowledge or hope

◆ Gain interest; refer to something you know is of interest to your reader or pay a compliment which leads easily into the first points of your letter plan.

Avoid overuse of phrases such as:

> We respectfully acknowledge receipt of
>
> I have to acknowledge with thanks
>
> I note the contents of your letter
>
> Referring to your communication dated...
>
> With reference to your letters of 15th ult. and 20th idem.

Ending a letter

The *final paragraphs* should specify the action. If your reader or readers have to do something, state exactly who, when, and what, and make it as easy for them to do as you can.

Make it clear what *happens next*. Are you going to write again? Are you expecting a reply? Is the matter closed?

Use a *friendly* tone. The best way of achieving this is to use a special, non-standard expression, perhaps something private between you and your reader, or refer to some common knowledge. If you cannot use an exclusive phrase, use a short one, such as 'Best wishes'. When you are trying to be friendly and polite, there is no value in using an 'off-the-shelf' phrase that is cumbersome.

Avoid *'Do not hesitate'*. It is too long and hackneyed to be personal. So, when you want to write, 'In the event of any further difficulty please do not hesitate to contact me', which is a good message, it is better to leave out 'Do not hesitate to'.

Avoid overuse of other phrases such as:

> We look forward to the favour of your instructions
>
> Thanking you in advance
>
> Assuring you of our best attention at all times
>
> Regretting our inability to be of service in this matter
>
> Trusting we may be favoured with
>
> Awaiting a favourable reply
>
> Your attention to this matter is urgently required.

Most of these endings are neither courteous nor efficient. If you want a quick reply, give a date, and say why you need it by that date, eg. for a meeting. This helps the reader to give your letter priority.

When signing off a letter to a close friend, all the writer has to do is put 'Yours' or 'Love', followed by the name usually used with the friend. The more common 'Yours sincerely' should only be used when the writer wants to be more formal. 'Yours faithfully' is used when the writer began the letter without giving a name, as in 'Dear Sir or Madam'. It is simply a question of how the writer began the letter, not how well the writer knows the reader. Capital letters in 'sincerely' or 'faithfully' are unconventional.

Type your name under your signature, and title (Dr, Mrs, etc.) and occupation, if it is relevant, unless you gave this information at the top of the letter; to do so is good public relations and helps your reader in formulating a reply.

Avoid postscripts as they indicate poor planning; in fact, some say that PS stands for 'planning sketchily'.

Memoranda

Memoranda are internal communications that are addressed to one person or a number of people about a specific subject. They provide the opportunity to improve communication between staff. It is important, therefore, that memoranda are eye-catching. If memoranda are monotonous in style and are sent too frequently they will not be read.

The following are some key points to bear in mind when sending memoranda:

1.   Make the main point at the beginning.

2.   Only give essential information.

3.   Write simply; do not use authoritarian language.

4.   Use headings to direct the reader to specific issues.

Remember, as with letters, memoranda should be planned before you begin writing.

Short reports

In nursing, writing a report has traditionally been associated with recording the patient's progress. More recently, however, as a result of managerial demands, organisational needs and professional accountability, report writing has taken on a wider meaning. The dictionary definitions of 'report' are interesting:

An account brought by one person to another, especially of some matters specially investigated

and

A formal statement of the result of an investigation, or any matter on which definite information is required, made by some person or body instructed or required to do so.

Nurses may be instructed to produce a report on a particular subject or they may want to produce a report on their own initiative, eg. following the introduction of a new standard of nursing practice from the UKCC which has implications for future local practice and resources. Reports can be short or long but on the whole they should be concise and precise. They are written to record, to inform and to recommend. The most important questions that a report writer must ask her/himself are:

◆ Why am I writing this report?

◆ Who is the intended audience?

◆ What is relevant and irrelevant?

If a manager or chief executive of a trust has asked for a particular report to be written it is important to clarify on what aspect the manager wants the nurse to concentrate. With the emphasis on evidence-based health care, recommendations need to be backed up with rationale and any relevant research references. An effective report should have a statement of purpose, under the heading 'Terms of reference', 'Purpose' or 'Introduction'. Such a statement helps subsequent readers and report writers to update and follow on where the previous writer has finished.

The key factors of an effective report are as follows

1. *Structure:* Structure is the framework within which ideas are expressed. A report can be structured through the use of headings and sub-headings. Structure also includes the sequence of points, paragraphing and numbering.

2. *Headings:* Headings give the reader an accurate guide as to what is in the text beneath. Vague headings such as 'General' or 'Other facts' are of little use. To help the reader find a particular section quickly, the headings and subheadings should be in a logical order.

3. *Sequence:* The purpose of the report should come first, perhaps under the heading 'Introduction'. The evidence should come next, divided under suitable headings. The writer should then pass judgement on the evidence, under 'Conclusions' or 'Discussion'. Finally, under 'Recommendations', the report should state what ought to happen next. If the reader is likely to read the conclusions and recommendations before the evidence, it may save time to set them out in that order, ie. 'Introduction', 'Conclusions', 'Recommendations' and, finally, 'Evidence'.

4. *Paragraphs:* Readers can more easily follow stages in an argument if each stage is in a separate paragraph. At least three paragraphs per side of A4 are reasonable, but sometimes more than six are necessary. A good test of whether a paragraph is a unified stage is whether it is possible to devise an accurate heading for it.

5. *Numbering:* It is convenient to number all the headings so that people can refer to particular sections in the document when on the telephone or at meetings. Arabic numerals are the easiest to recognise. The best method of numbering sub-headings is by using the 'decimal' system: 1.1, 1.2, 1.3, 1.4 and so on.

6. *Conclusions:* These should be carefully written, in a clear and concise style. It is often easier to list the conclusions and then go on to add a summary of the key evidence which supports the conclusions. There may well be several possibilities or options to consider and supportive evidence should be given for each alternative.

7. **Recommendations:** These should be kept separate from the conclusions and include personal preferences, economic considerations and professional advice. Keeping recommendations simple or subdividing them in to short- and long-term strategies aids quick referencing and rapid use.

8. **Appendices:** These should contain any relevant technical or professional information such as sections from reports and statistical or other research data. A glossary of technical nursing and medical terms used may be a helpful inclusion at either the end or start of the report.

Finally, reports come to life and are more readable and interesting if colour photographs and diagrams are used.

Summary

Patient information can be recorded and reported more effectively if nurses bear in mind the importance of interpersonal communication skills. Presenting information in an objective, accurate and clear manner reduces the likelihood of it being misunderstood or ignored. It is important for nurses to reflect on how effective their interpersonal skills are and how well they are assessing and interpreting the needs of the patient. Often, more time spent listening to what patients have to say will avoid embarrassing inaccuracies in nursing records and reports.

3

Legal and ethical implications

Introduction

Good nursing care is your best defence against being sued for malpractice. However, if you do get into difficulties then clear and accurate documentation of the nursing care provided will be your best defence in the courtroom.

Documentation of care has become synonymous with care itself. If you fail to document care the court will probably assume that you failed to provide care and/or that you are an unprofessional practitioner. The following are some basic charting guidelines which govern documentation, regardless format of records or charts used.

Accuracy: Make sure that what you are writing down is a true reflection of what you wish to happen or has happened, or shows concrete and accurate evidence of the use of the nursing process.

Relevance: Relevant entries need to include information about the patient's history, nursing assessment, nursing problems or concerns, care plans, interventions (either physician or nurse-initiated), a diary of what happened and reference to audit or evaluation of nursing care. Information relating to transfer or discharge home should be started as soon as possible and should include relevant forms and contacts with community services. Evidence of continuity of care from one setting to the next is important, especially when dealing with vulnerable patients such as chronically sick or older people.

Completeness: Following on from relevance is the importance of making sure that a record contains all the pertinent points and covers the whole spectrum of nursing care that has been provided for the patient. All records should be completed as soon as possible after care delivery. Often, nursing records read well on first contact with the patient, but then deteriorate. Sometimes, assessments are not followed up or repeated when the patient's condition changes. Frequency of charting is often determined by local policy, the patient's condition,, and the time available for writing up records.

The patient's nursing records should cover not only the stages of the nursing process and discharge planning but also the effects of all health interventions and the patient's progress throughout her/his period of care.

Alertness: Do not allow yourself to become complacent about your documentation. Many unexpected things happen (probably when you least expect them) not only directly to the patient but also in relation to the context and environment of care. Some of these incidents or events may not fit into the normal pattern of recording or system used for documentation. If concerned or worried about a particular matter then keep a written record of it.

Conciseness: Nurses often feel that they have to describe or discuss a situation in depth. This can sometimes lead to a lengthy and wordy account. When documenting care, try to be economical with words, use short sentences, and be succinct and precise. Get to the point and avoid using irrelevant details that increase length without providing useful infomation.

Timeliness: Records should be suitable for the purpose for which they have been designed. The timing of an event or incident is important. Therefore, whenever making an entry, think carefully about the relevance and accuracy of the time things should have or have occurred.

Legibility and construction

Poor handwriting, spelling, an unnatural order of events and the use of inappropriate words are some of the main causes of illegibility. Such errors may lead courts to conclude that professional communication is poor and that the documentation is a reflection of the quality of care.

As the nursing record is a legal document it is often used in court. Nurses may be asked to defend what they have written and give reasons for the way in which the information has been recorded. Statistically, however, the standard of records and record keeping by nurses, midwives and health visitors is poor.

In the UKCC's professional conduct hearings, nursing records are usually used as evidence for accuracy of events surrounding a case as they are more reliable than a nurse's recollection of what has occurred. Therefore, nurses should keep accurate records not only for legal reasons but also for professional credibility and survival on the UKCC's Register.

Charting guidelines

All nurses must familiarise themselves with the UKCC's *Standards for Records and Record Keeping* (see *Chapter 4)* And be aware of local policies and guidelines.

Before writing entries into records make sure you have identified the correct clinical record. If you make a mistake, it is best to draw a clear line through it, date and sign (using full signature) and write 'error'. Never obliterate with ink or white-out correction fluid. Obliterations that do not permit a reader to see the text underneath are suspicious and raise questions about the reason for the obliteration.

Always write notes in indelible ink using every line. It is important to avoid leaving gaps between entries as this will reduce the likelihood of someone adding false information at a later stage. Record the patient's name and identification number on every page or chart you use. Entries should be clearly dated stating the day, month and year. It is also advisable to include the time of the entry, especially when charting periodically during a shift. Do not document in advance or allow someone else to document care that you have given. An exception to this is in an emergency situation, such as cardiopulmonary resuscitation, when one nurse may document the care given by many people during the event.

The type of information that needs to be documented

◆ The nursing interventions you have carried out

◆ Doctors' prescribed measures that you carry out

◆ The patient's health-related behaviour such as physical signs, actions and reactions

◆ The patient's verbal response (always use direct quotations and describe the emotional tone)

◆ The patient's specific responses to therapies and care given during your involvement

◆ Visits and consultations (including telephone conversations) by doctors and other members of the health care team

◆ If you question a doctor's order, document your question and how it was answered; include the discussion and the date/time of the conversation

◆ Relatives' and significant others' questions and comments, especially if they are contentious.

All nursing records must be signed at the end of the entry, and subsequent entries if additional notes have been added during the same shift or home visit. Student nurses and health care assistants/ auxiliaries should record their own specific contribution and sign the record, stating their title, eg. student or auxiliary.

There have been cases where registered or primary nurses have signed for care or observations carried out by others. This is not a recommended practice. Remember that you will be held responsible for the completeness and accuracy of everything that you have signed. If you have to record care of which you lack first-hand knowledge, write, 'patient bathed by Auxiliary Jones, who reports that the patient has back pain'. If an incident occurs involving one of your patients it is advisable to record what happened in two places, ie. the progress notes and the incident form. If you are concerned about a patient's welfare, safety or environment of care, it is advisable to record all your concerns, relevant conversations, letters and telephone calls.

In cases where you recall omitting important information that you should have recorded at the time, use the next available space and start with the heading, 'Addendum to nurse's note of day, month and time'.

Accurate documentation will increase your credibility in disputes between yourself and a doctor, senior nurse, general manager or other member of a health care team. Lack of documentation does not always imply negligence, but it will be more difficult to prove your case without it. A common expression is 'If it wasn't charted it wasn't done'.

Litigation

Record keeping that complies with established standards of care is a legitimate form of self-protection against litigation and can help when determining liability.

Common types of litigation involving nurses

The objectives of good record keeping outlined above are a mark of professional practice and have two further important functions:

(a) They may prevent a nurse from becoming involved in litigation. For example, a patient may complain that a nurse did not carry out a procedure but if the records show that the procedure was carried out and that the records were made at the time of, or shortly after, the event, then they are likely to persuade the patient's legal adviser that there is little point in bringing a case.

(b) In the unfortunate event of a nurse being caught up in litigation then accurate, contemporaneous records may constitute an excellent defence.

The main involvement of nurses in the litigation process is in respect of their own accidents. This section does not deal with this type of case except to remind nurses that the best record of an accident is an early note in the accident book.

The two most important areas of legal liability for a nurse relate to procedures carried out without proper consent and negligent treatment.

Why would anyone want to sue you?

If a patient claims that things have gone wrong, eg. she/he suffered permanent bladder problems after being catheterised incompetently, she/he does not have an automatic right to compensation. To recover damages she/he must be able to show that she/he has a good legal case and, sometimes, she/he may have to go to court. Normally, the patient will sue your employer in which case you may have to be a witness. Although you may have made the mistake your employer will normally be legally responsible for your actions.

Legal duty to take care

An NHS patient, whether of a trust, GP fundholder, health authority or ordinary GP, does not have a contract with the health provider: the provider and staff offer a service on a statutory basis and owe a duty to everyone treated to carry out the work properly. The same duty applies to the nurse who provides 'Good Samaritan' treatment, ie. voluntary care given in an emergency.

A hospital is responsible for its own actions (eg. did it hire a suitably qualified agency nurse, was there a safe system of work?); and it is responsible for the actions of its own staff. (In some cases it may be responsible for agency staff.) This is called *vicarious responsibility*.

A disturbing new development is for trusts to attempt to recover from a staff member damages it has had to pay out because of the staff member's negligence (an indemnity). Nurses need to take advice about this and make sure that they are adequately insured.

In the private sector patients make a contract with the hospital and if this is broken (eg. a particular level of service was not maintained as promised) they can sue for damages. The NHS guarantees no particular level of service — *The Patient's Charter* does not have the force of law and a trust or health authority cannot be sued if it does not keep to a promised service level.

What is the standard of care required?

In a case relating to a road accident, the defendant will lose if she/he has driven her/his car below the standards of the reasonable man. For a case that does not involve any special skill, negligence in law means: some failure to do some act which a reasonable man in the circumstances would do; and if that failure or doing of that act results in injury, then there is a cause of action. How do you test whether this act or failure is negligent? In an ordinary case it is generally said, that you judge that by the action of the person in the street. She/he is the ordinary person. In one case it has been said that you judge it by the conduct of the person on the top of a Clapham omnibus. He is the ordinary person.

Nursing is different as, it involves the use of special skill or competence. The test to see if a nurse was negligent is not the test of the person on top of a Clapham omnibus. It is the standard test of the ordinary skilled nurse exercising and professing to have a special skill. A nurse need not possess the highest expert skill. It is well-established law that it is sufficient if the nurse has exercised the ordinary skill of an ordinary competent nurse.

What if the nurse is covering for someone else?

The standard is job not person specific. A nurse will be judged by the standards of the job she/he is doing and not her/his own standards. For example, if asked to stand in as first assistant she/he will be judged as an experienced first assistant and not a stand-in. After all, the patient is entitled to proper treatment from appropriately qualified staff. (It would be different if the operation was an emergency and had to proceed quickly with whatever staff were at hand.)

What if there are differences of opinion as to what is the right (non-negligent) way to act?

Take the important case of Mr Bolam (Bolam *vs* Friern Hospital Management Committee [1957]). He was injured when electro-convulsive therapy (ECT) treatment caused him to have such violent fits that his femur heads were driven through the cups of his pelvis. At that time (1954) there were three recognised restraint regimes during ECT:

Treatment A = ECT= muscle relaxant

Treatment B = ECT+ restraint by nurse

Treatment C = ECT+ physyical restraint

Mr Bolam's doctors had chosen treatment model B.The doctors were not negligent in choosing B as they had made a genuine choice. In retrospect, a better choice would have been A (now the standard approach but then only just coming into vogue) but a court will not criticise a nurse or other health professional for working according to the acceptable standards of the time.

It is important to note that if there is a difference of opinion, neither is necessarily wrong — it is not like driving where there is only one way to turn right at a junction (as prescribed by *The Highway Code*). The driver who turns right 'wrongly' is clearly negligent; the nurse who chooses one of a range of approaches is not negligent.

The Bolam case produced the Bolam test which continues to this day:

(a) Medical negligence occurs where there is a duty of care and the plaintiff can show, on a balance of probabilities (ie. that it is more likely than not), that the defendant nurse has fallen below the ordinary skill of a reasonably skilled and experienced competent practitioner in the field.

(b) The test is against the nurse practising in her/his particular field of medicine (eg. CPN against CPN as opposed to CPN against practice nurse).

(c) When the standard of skill is an issue (as is often the case with medical negligence) the defendant nurse's case will be judged against the standards of the UKCC and professional associations.

The role of expert opinion

Some medical negligence cases are tried on the facts alone, eg. it is agreed by all parties that before procedure A the nurse should have given drug B. The nurse claims to have done so but there is no record and the patient denies that she/he was injected.

Most cases which go to trial involve a dispute over the correct medical approach, with experts arguing as to the appropriateness of the diagnosis made, the treatment given or the advice offered. As explained above, to win such a case the plaintiff would normally have to show that no responsible nurse would have acted (or failed to act) as the defendant nurse did, and in order to do this the allegation must have the support of expert nursing opinion. Experts called in medical negligence cases tend to be leaders in their field, impartially available to plaintiffs and defendants alike, who are currently in practice or recently retired.

The role of causation

Consider a patient with advanced cardiovascular disease refusing to give up a heavy smoking habit and who is already a bilateral amputee. He is prescribed a blood-thinning agent but by error this is given in insufficient strength. After suffering a stroke, his medication is revised but he continues to have strokes and eventually dies. It would be hard to prove that the mistake played a part in his death as he was already beyond effective treatment. Mistakes can occur despite the best possible training and guidelines. However, few errors can be legally linked to a poor result. To do this the patient would have to show, on the balance of probabilities, that the error was legally negligent and, again on the balance of probabilities, that the negligence led to that poor result. The progress of illness is such that it is often difficult to demonstrate the *good* that treatment does, let alone the *harm* that poor treatment causes.

With the increase in responsibility that results from the traditional roles of nurses extending into new areas of diagnosis and treatment comes the increased possibility of nurses being in the firing line. The difficulties of proving a case, as outlined above, mean that very few medical accidents culminate in court cases. Good nursing practice, allied with good record keeping, should be sufficient protection to avoid legal problems.

Factors that increase legal risk

There are several factors that nurses should guard against if they are to protect themselves from accusations of poor professional record keeping:

1. Content of records not in line with UKCC and health care service standards and guidelines.
2. Content does not reflect patient needs.
3. Content does not include descriptions of situations that are out of the ordinary.
4. Lack of detail regarding nursing assessments, observations, interventions and evaluations.
5. Poor progress notes — content not logical, timely or in a chronological sequence.
6. Incomplete or inconsistent content.
7. Content does not describe nursing care given and patients' responses.
8. Poorly recorded responses, of both themselves and their patients, to appropriate medical orders.
9. Different handwriting, white-out and obliterations suggestive of tampering.
10. Illegibility.

Ethical issues

There is no doubt that we are now living in an age of rapid change, with medical and technological discoveries reaching new frontiers. Some of these medical innovations will be of benefit to the whole population, whereas others will only focus on certain health needs. Unfortunately, such developments can be expensive and issues relating to who should benefit from them, what criteria should be used to assess priorities and how long treatment should be carried out often arise. Injuries and conditions that not so long ago would have resulted in a certain and fairly swift death can now be treated and, if not cured, at least held at bay.

Consumerism, with its emphasis on the role of the receiver of health care services, has resulted in the patient having a more open and questioning relationship with her/his doctor and nurse. No longer are patients expected to sit and wait for long periods without adequate explanation or accept decisions made for them by autocratic staff. Also, patients now have access to their health records.

Therefore, the keywords used in ethical discussions about patient care and documentation are: autonomy, freedom, rights, empowerment, privacy, access and confidentiality.

In order to make decisions efficiently and with the co-operation of others, nurses often follow conventional ethical principles. For example:

1. Nurses have an obligation to keep up-to-date, and be competent and accountable for their nursing care

2. Nurses have an obligation to the UKCC's standards of care and to 'care', 'protect' and 'honour' patients

3. The welfare of patients should be the nurse's primary concern

4. Nurses should be aware of their limitations

5. Nurses should not use their position to exploit patients

6. Nurses should be loyal to each other

7. Nurses should strive to work and cooperate with all members of the health care team

8. Nurses should follow the UKCC's (1992a) *Code of Professional Conduct* guidelines and, in relation to documentation, its *Standards for Records and Record Keeping* (see *Chapter 4).*

These principles summarise the fundamental points outlined in the UKCC's *Code of Professional Conduct* and highlight the common principles of nursing practice, which are consistent with more general philosophical ethical concepts. Such principles are used not only by nurses to justify their actions, but also by professional conduct committees and lawyers to evaluate nurses' behaviour.

'Flower' ethical grid

To help nurses develop their moral reasoning and decision-making in relation to ethical dilemmas, the construction of an ethical grid is proposed, similar to that outlined by Seedhouse (1988). This 'flower' grid has been adapted to include key ethical terms associated with documentation and is designed to act as an aide memoire or a model that can be used by nurses when faced with the ethical challenges of practice and, in particular, documentation issues (*Figure 3.1*).

Figure 3.1: Flower ethical grid

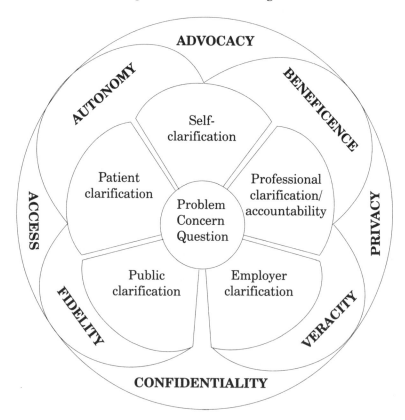

The central core of the model begins with the concern, problem or question that confronts the nurse. Surrounding this are five crucial clarifying areas or questions that the nurse should ask her/himself about the central core question:

1. *Self-clarification* — relates to questions about the values the nurse holds dear to her/his heart.

2. *Professional clarification and accountability* — relates to the standards and guidelines proposed by the UKCC. The nurse is accountable for her/his actions. Therefore, she/he must assess the issue in relation to this, ie. should she/he become involved in the situation?

3. *Employer clarification* — refers to the guidelines, directions, protocols, rules and regulations held by the nurse's employer.

4. *Patient clarification* — emphasises the importance of considering the patient's view, values and needs.

5. *Public clarification* — relates to society's current views on ethical issues such as euthanasia and abortion.

Surrounding these five questions are key ethical concerns relating to issues associated with records and record keeping. These are:

1. **Autonomy** — generally accepted as the respect we have for others as human beings that allows them to have control over their own lives.

2. **Beneficence** — the duty the nurse has to do good to others and by doing this to help them further their interests and avoid harm.

3. **Fidelity** — faithfulness and loyalty to the patient and her/his nursing care. This is the key foundation of the nurse/patient relationship.

4. **Veracity** — truth-telling and keeping promises.

5. **Advocacy** — once the nurse understands the patient's goals, hopes and fears, she/he must use her/his professional expertise and judgement to help the patient while respecting the patient's autonomy. Advocacy means acting for or on behalf of the patient with regard to her/his nursing and health needs.

6. **Privacy** — it is important that the nurse safeguards the patient's right to privacy by judiciously protecting information of a confidential nature. Privacy means being kept away from unnecessary public scrutiny.

7. **Confidentiality** — when a patient tells a nurse something in confidence it is important that she/he does not share it with anybody else unless the patient permits this. In some cases the patient may agree that certain information can be shared with other members of the health care team but no-one else. The nurse must clarify this before recording and reporting patient information. Also, it is important for the nurse to warn the patient that if she/he wants to reveal something that may compromise the nurse's position, eg. if the patient has committed a crime, then she/he may be unable to remain silent.

8. **Access** — usually refers to who should be allowed to, and how to, retrieve stored information. Patient information should be disseminated only on a need-to-know basis. Patients' right of access to information about themselves is enshrined in law in the Access to Medical Reports Act 1988 and the Access to Health Records Act 1990. The 1990 Act gives patients access to health records made after 1 November 1991 and to information recorded earlier this will help them to understand the later records. Computer records are subject to the Data Protection Act 1984, which gives legal protection to individuals against the misuse of personal information.

How to use the 'flower' ethical grid

An example core problem or question that the nurse may be faced with is as follows: a patient is indicating that he wants to know his diagnosis, in this case, cancer, but the relatives do not want him to be told. What should the nurse do?

First, following the grid's pattern, the nurse must seek to clarify more carefully and succinctly the exact nature of the problem. The nurse must then carefully consider the situation by reviewing her/his personal view of the problem, professional responsibilities and accountability, employer and public issues and, finally, the patient's wishes and needs. In this case the nurse may feel that there is sufficient evidence to support the patient.

Consideration of key ethical concepts surrounding the first five clarification points lends more support to the patient being told his diagnosis. For example: veracity supports the notion of telling the truth about the diagnosis; autonomy means that the patient has a right to know his diagnosis; beneficence relates to the nurse's role in avoiding upset to the patient by not allowing him to know what is happening to him; and fidelity suggests that the nurse/ patient relationship should be based on honesty.

The nurse must finally consider the concepts contained in the outer ring of the grid. Advocacy, for example, may help the nurse to view the poroblem from the patient's perspective, ie. not knowing his diagnosis; access may help the nurse to consider what the key blocks are to the patient knowing his diagnosis; and confidentiality relates to how this information should be conveyed.

It is important to stress that this ethical grid is only a guide to clarifying ethical problems or questions. It is not a substitute for the nurse actively participating in further team disscussions and ethical interdisciplinary reviews and case conferences.

Consent

The requirement of informed consent is a legal protection of a person's moral right to personal autonomy. When a consent form is signed it should indicate that the patient has made an informed and free decision to undergo a procedure, treatment or specific nursing therapy. There are various aspects to informed consent. First, a decision is only informed if the person has been given all the information that she/he might consider helpful in reaching the decision. Second, the decision should be made freely and without pressure or coercion from others. Third, consent must be obtained from the patient/client before any form of treatment can commence, except, of course, in emergency situations. Fourth, consent may be given only for a particular time span or the extent of action proposed on the informed consent document.

Although consent for medical treatment is primarily the

responsibility of a physician, a nurse may be held responsible for not detecting that all the elements of informed consent had been met. This is particularly relevant if the consent relates to a nursing therapy or treatment. Therefore, if nurses discover any of the problems listed below they should report their concerns immediately and record their observations and actions in the nursing records:

1. The nurse detects that the patient does not seem to understand the procedure, treatment or risks.

2. The patient states that she/he has not signed her/his consent form.

3. There is no signature on the consent form.

4. The doctor says that she/he has not had time to explain the proposed treatment to the patient.

5. Someone else has signed the consent form on behalf of the patient when it was inappropriate to do so (eg. the patient is old enough to do it for her/himself).

6. There has been a considerable time span since the patient signed the form, or the proposed treatment as recorded on the consent form has changed significantly.

7. The patient has reversed her/his decision and has decided against treatment.

Meeting the criteria of an informed and free consent is difficult in health care settings today but it is important that the nurse is sensitive to and aware of this aspect of documentation.

Privacy, confidentiality and access to nursing records

With the rapid developments in computer-based record keeping and increasing technological possibilities for the electronic sharing of patient information, there are growing concerns in relation to the use and disclosure of private and confidential information.

Patient privacy

When trying to maintain confidentiality of patient information, it is important for the key nurse in charge of the patient's nursing care to think carefully about which members of the nursing and non-nursing team should be allowed access to the information in the patient's records. There may be some personal aspects of the patient's case history which should be accessible only to those very close to the patient. For example, nursing assistants and some agency and bank staff may only be involved in peripheral tasks for the patients. In this case, accessible information should be limited to that which is relevant to nursing the patient during the shift and disseminated on a need-to-know basis only.

Anyone with access to patient information should be reminded of her/his responsibility to protect the patient's privacy. For example, casual conversations in canteens are frequent sources of privacy violations. Releasing patient information into a network system for the purposes of transfer and discharge can also lead to the inadvertent sharing of information. Carelessness with sensitive patient information can have tremendous economic and social ramifications for patients, families and society, eg. in the case of patients with human immunodeficiency virus or aquired immunodeficiency syndrome (HIV/AIDS). Release of sensitive information could deny patient groups health insurance cover or access to other resources. Policies and procedures for blocking or coding sensitive data so that they do not routinely appear on charts or computer screens is essential if we are to prevent the inadvertent transmission of such information.

Paper-based patient record systems may permit unauthorised, unnecessary and undetected access. Therefore, it could be argued that the introduction of sophisticated computer codes would make patient information more secure.

Health care professionals have adopted ethical codes that address the key issues of privacy and confidentiality. Unfortunately, many people who collect or access a patient's health care information are not health care professionals and therefore they also need to be bound by an ethical code and receive regular training in ethics and privacy issues.

The Institute of Health Informatics states that: 'There is no single solution to the issue of the security of the clinical record, rather, there is a set of "core" principles' (Gries and Currell, 1995). Of all these, patient consent and co-operation are probably the most crucial. Another way of ensuring that the patient remains in control is by encouraging greater use of patient-held health care records. The concept of information being stored on an easy-to-carry computer card which can be used when and where required is in the process of being developed. There are three major aspects of privacy: the patient's / client's right to privacy; protection of information; and access to records.

Nurses are ethically bound to hold all information in confidence. Only in exceptional circumstances, such as child or elder abuse, should a nurse disclose patient/client information to other interested and relevant individuals. Apart from these exceptions, the nurse should always consider the wellbeing, safety and rights of the patient/client when determining the dissemination of confidential information.

With the emphasis on multidisciplinary health care teams it is important that nurses share relevant aspects of the data they have collected. They should, however, do this carefully because of the possible misuses to whichsuch information can be put. For example, health records are a rich source of research and quality audit. Patients'/clients' consent must always be gained before their records can be used for any purpose other than helping them with their particular health care problems. If patient information is to be used for such purposes, anonymity must be observed at all times.

Patient/client information should be disseminated on a need-to-know basis only. From a nursing perspective, all nurses involved in the care of a patient must have access to all information that affects the patient's care.

Confidentiality

The concept of confidentiality goes back to the time of Hippocrates and beyond. Initially, it related to the doctor/patient relationship but now it also relates to the nurse/patient relationship and the importance of nurses preserving the information they know about a patient/client.

Clause 10 of the UKCC's (1992a) *Code of Professional Conduct* addresses the subject of confidentiality directly when it states that:

As a registered nurse, midwife or health visitor, you are personally accountable for your practice and in the exercise of your professional accountability must... protect all confidential information concerning patients and clients obtained in the course of professional practice and make disclosures only with consent, where required by the order of a court or where you can justify disclosure in the wider public interest.

Nursing information about patients can be recorded in a variety of ways. Some of these form part of the recognised written record or may be additional sheets of information relating to conversations with the patient or even audiovisual material. In some situations access to the records of patients/clients may be necessary to help in the education of nursing students, eg. care studies and care plans based on contacts with patients/clients. Therefore, it is important to stress to students the importance of confidentiality and anonymity.

Whatever type of record is being used or developed about a particular patient, it is important to check with the patient that their permission has been granted and that the record is not being used for anything other than the purpose for which it was intended.

Computer records will probably replace manual records over the next few years. It is important, however, that the principles relating to written records are transferred to computer-based systems. The Data Protection Act 1984 gives legal protection to individuals against the misuse of personal information; the Access to Medical Reports Act 1988 gives right of access to information; and the Access to Health Records 1990 gives patients access to their health records made after 1 November, 1991.

The British Medical Association (BMA) encourages doctors to give patients access to all health information held about them, unless the doctor believes it deleterious to the patient's health to do so, or unless the confidentiality of other people might be compromised. Such advice also applies to nurses about access to patients' nursing records.

The confidentiality of and access to health information about minors and legal dependants is of concern to nurses as these groups are particularly vulnerable to violations of confidentiality and privacy. Mental health legislation allows persons appointed on the patient's behalf to exercise a right of access. Surprisingly, the age of the patient is not relevant to access. If patients are minors and capable of giving consent, parents must have their consent to apply for access to their records (BMA, 1993). Minors may wish to keep some matters they have raised with their doctors secret from their parents. Parents are, at present, helpless to do anything about this except put pressure on their children to agree to let them see the records.

In conclusion, nurses are advocates for patients. They must restrict access to patient information and realise that such information should be disseminated on a need-to-know basis only. The overriding goal must be to protect the patient from unauthorised and unnecessary invasions of privacy. Finally, patients have the right to view their own clinical health records. Nursing documentation, therefore, should be written in the knowledge that the patient may one day want to read it.

Advance directives

The most common example of an advance directive is the written will. Throughout history, wills have been viewed as the efficient legal way of disposing with a person's property after her/his death. However, more recently, they have been adapted to express a person's wishes with regard to future medical treatment.

Keatings and Smith (1995) define an advance directive as:

A document made and signed by a mentally competent adult detailing specific medical treatments that are to be administered or withheld in the event that the maker later becomes incapable of expressing such wishes owing to mental or physical illness (eg. Alzheimer's disease, coma).

In 1994, the House of Lords Select Committee on Medical Ethics called for a code of practice on advance directives for health professionals, including nurses. This resulted in the BMA publishing such a code in 1995 in collaboration with the medical and nursing Royal Colleges (BMA, 1995).

This Code points out that:

◆ Although not binding on health professional,s advance statements deserve thorough consideration and respect

◆ Where valid and applicable, advance directives (refusals) must be followed

◆ Health professionals consulted by people wishing to formulate an advance statement or directive should take all reasonable steps to provide accurate factual information about the treatment options and their implications

◆ Where an unknown and incapacitated patient presents for treatment some checks should be made cncerning the validity of any directive refusing life-prolonging treatment. In all cases, it is vital to check that the statement or refusal presented is that of the patient being treated and has not been withdrawn

◆ If the situation is not identical to that described in the advance statement or refusal, treatment providers may still be guided by the general spirit of the statement if this is evident. It is advisable to contact any person nominated by the patient as well as the GP to clarify the patient's wishes. If there is doubt as to what the patient intended, the law requires the exercise of a best interests judgement

◆ If an incapacitated person is known to have had sustained and informed objections to all or some treatment, even though these have not been formally recorded, health professionals may not be justified in proceeding. This applies even in an emergency

◆ If witnessed and made at a time when the patient was competent and informed, such objections may constitute an oral advance directive. Health professionals will need to consider how much evidence is available about the patient's decision and how convincing it seems. The entire health care team can contribute to this process

◆ In the absence of any indication of the patient's wishes, there is a common law duty to give appropriate treatment to incapacitated patients when the treatment is clearly in their best interests.

According to Molloy and Mepham (1993), there are two types of advance directives:

1. An institutional directive which states the treatments wanted or not under any given circumstances. These statements can be as general or as specific as desired. The more specific they are, however,the easier they are for nurses, doctors and family to follow

2. A proxy directive which nominates another person (the proxy) to make decisions for the patient's health care if the patient has become incompetent. This proxy has the ability to make health care decisions in much the same way as a power of attorney does for financial matters.

Certain pressure groups such as The Voluntary Euthanasia Society proposes a 'Let me decide' health care directive which combines both an institutional and a proxy directive. According to the BMA (1995), there are various types of advanced directives:

◆ A statement reflecting an individual's aspirations and preferences. this can help health professionals identify how the person would like to be treated without binding him/her to that course of action, if it conflicts with professional judgement

◆ A statement of the general beliefs and aspects of life which an individual values. this provides a summary of individual responses to a list of questions about a person's past and present wishes and future desires. It makes no specific request or refusal but attempts to give a biographical portrait of the individual as an aid to deciding what she/he would want

◆ A statement which names another person who should be consulted at the time a decision has to be made. the views expressed by that named person should reflect what the patient would want. this can supplement and clarify the intended scope of a written statement but the named person's views are presently not legally binding in England and Wales. In Scotland, the powers of a tutor dative may cover such eventualities

◆ A clear instruction refusing some or all medical procedures (advance directive). made by a competent adult, this does, in certain circumstances, have legal force

◆ A statement which, rather than refusing any particular treatment, specifies a degree of irreversible deterioration (such as a diagnosis of persistent vegetative state) after which no life-sustaining treatment should be given. For adults, this again can have legal force

◆ A combination of the above, including requests, refusals and the nomination of a representative. Those sections expressing clear refusal may have legal force in the case of adult patients.

The nurse should be aware that an advance statement can be a written document, a witnessed oral statement, a signed printed card, a smart card or a note of a discussion recorded in the patient's file. Only a clear refusal of a particular treatment by an adult has potential legal force (BMA, 1995).

It is important that the presence or, in some cases, absence of an advance directive is documented in the nursing records. If a patient has prepared an advance directive, everyone, including her/his doctors, must be made aware of it. Also, it would be advisable to record its location and obtain a copy for the patient's records.

If a patient informs you that she/he does not want to be resuscitated, this statement must be documented. Nursing documentation should reflect patients' rights, in order to facilitate informed decision-making regarding advance directives. Any change in patient intent must be recorded.

'Not for resuscitation' orders

Sometimes patients' notes are marked 'Not for resuscitation' (NFR), 'Do not resuscitate' (DNR) or another term which indicates that cardiopulmonary resuscitation (CPR) should not be carried out. This ˈause a great deal of anxiety for nurses. The UKCC (see *'ards for Records and Record Keeping; Chapter 4)* emphasises ˈportance of :

◆ Accurately reflecting wishes of the patient
◆ Accurately reflecting the wishes of the patient's next of kin or significant others
◆ The decision 'not to' being based on clinical grounds by the relevant medical staff
◆ Entering such opinions and decisions in the medical record which should be signed and dated by the responsible registered medical practitioner
◆ The whole health care team, including nurses, being part of the decision
◆ The entry in the medical record being located easily and quickly
◆ The inclusion of a time limit after which the decision must be reviewed
◆ The nursing staff transferring the decision into the nursing record only *after* it has been recorded in the medical record.

If a nurse does not initiate emergency CPR when ' NFR' is not written in the notesd it could be argued that she/he is making a medical decision for which she/he is not qualified. On the other hand, if the nurse ignores the letters 'NFR' and starts resuscitation procedures,she/he would have to justify her/his decision. Usually, CPR is not indicated in cases of terminal irreversible illness where death is not unexpected or where prolonged resuscitation efforts would be futile. In these circumstances resuscitation may represent a violation of an individual's right to die with dignity (Creighton, 1986).

It is therefore important to stress that nurses should always be involved in discussion about NFR orders and record such decisions clearly and carefully.

4

Documentation standards

The importance of standards

The accountability of health care institutions, physicians and nurses has changed dramatically over the past few years. This is largely due to *The Patient's Charter* (Department of Health, 1991) which highlighted the importance of patient and client feedback and their involvement in their health care. The increasing number of successful legal claims and settlements out of court have made health care providers, both individuals and institutions, fully aware of their responsibility for patients' safety.

As a consequence of increased litigation, health care providers have developed risk management programmes and quality assurance systems as methods of protecting, maintaining and assuring high quality care for patients. Quality assurance is the method by which performance of care is evaluated for effectiveness. Standards for appropriate care are established and provide the basis upon which potential risk can be assessed. Following this, measures to reduce risk can be introduced. Quality assurance is the foundation of any risk management programme. In nursing terms, quality assurance is the systematic process of evaluating the quality of nursing care given in a particular nursing setting or place where nurses work. It involves: setting standards; determining criteria to meet the standards; evaluating how well the criteria have been met; making plans for change based on evaluation; and implementation.

In the same way that many standards influence and govern nursing responsibilities and nursing practice, standards also influence and govern the documentation of nursing practice.

By definition, a standard is a measure or statement to which other similar things should conform. Its value is ultimately determined by evidence of its consistent use and evaluation. A nursing standard is no different than any other health care standard that is set by an institution or health care provider. It should describe the quality, characteristics, properties or performance requirements of an aspect of nursing practice.

Sources of standards

The standards governing nursing documentation derive from several sources:

◆ The UKCC

◆ The Department of Health

◆ Policies and procedures to which health care providers subscribe

◆ Documents generated by professional organisations

◆ Research- and evidence-based health care.

Standards are influenced by public concern, court cases, professional conduct hearings and other sources of professional and union activity.

Nurses need documentation standards to provide direction and guidance for sound record-keeping practices and appropriate reporting procedures. When standards are made they need to be clear so that nursing colleagues and other health care professionals, including quality assurance reviewers, can easily follow them.

The UKCC's *Standard for Records and Record Keeping* was first published in 1993; it has been reproduced at the end of this chapter. It is divided into several sections: the purpose of records; the importance of records; key features of standards for records; ethical aspects; recording decisions on resuscitation; essential elements; and various notes relating to patient and client access, shared records and overall principles. To meet the standards set out in its document, the UKCC links them with its *Code of Professional Conduct* (UKCC, 1992a). It is therefore expected that all nurses will be judged by their actions and ability to:

(1)   Act always in such a manner as to promote and safeguard the

interests and well-being of patients and clients

(2) Ensure that no action or omission on your part, or within your sphere of responsibility, is detrimental to the interests, conditions or safety of patients and clients

(10) Protect all confidential information concerning patients and clients obtained in the course of professional practice and make disclosures only with consent, where required by the order of a court or where you can justify disclosure in the wider public interest (UKCC, 1992a).

The *Code of Professional Conduct* contains 16 clauses altogether, but these three are the most relevant to record keeping.

In *Standards for Record and Record Keeping,* the UKCC states that there is substantial evidence to indicate that inadequate and inappropriate record keeping is leading to poor continuity of care, failures in communication between staff and inadequate protection from error.

Setting standards for records and record keeping promotes vital elements of consumer satisfaction. For example, standards reflect comsumer rights and the outcomes which nurses are trying to achieve and which patients expect. With regard to nurses, standards provide: guidelines for professional accountabilty; promotion of nursing satisfaction by defining acceptable protocols for nursing practice; outcome criteria so that nursing care can be evaluated; and clarification of the unique contribution that nurses make to health care.

The UKCC's annual analysis of its professional conduct statistics emphasizes the importance of documentation standards and the need for accurate record keeping. *Table 4.1* shows the frequency of occurrence of certain types of practice-based offences during the period April 1996–March 1997. Failure to keep accurate records of report incidents comes third in the overall table.

Table 4.1: UKCC professional conduct statistics, April 1996–March 1997		
Type of offence	**Number**	**%**
Physical/verbal abuse of patient/clients	166	31.09
Failure/inappropriate attention to basic needs	64	11.99
Failure to keep accurate records or reports	51	9.55
Miscellaneous	48	8.99
Unsafe clinical practice	29	5.43
Sexual harrassment of colleagues	21	3.93
Physical/verbal abuse of other staff	19	3.56
Patient abuse (other)	19	3.56
Other dishonesty	16	3.00
Abuse of management authority	15	2.81
Other drug related	14	2.62
Sleeping on duty	11	2.06
Failure to collaborate with colleagues	11	2.06
Unfit for duty — drink/drugs	10	1.87
Theft from patients/clients	9	1.69
Sexual abuse of patients/clients	9	1.69
False claim to register	6	1.12
Misadministration of drug	5	0.94
Theft from employers	3	0.56
Misappropriation of drugs	3	0.56
Poor practice	2	0.37
Breaches of confidentiality	2	0.37
Failure to communicate/seek consent	1	0.19
Abuse of patients/clients — drugs	0	0.00
Total	534	100.00

Key standards

The collection of data about the nursing care of a patient should show:

1. The type and quality of the nurse's assessment of the patient. This should include information relating to the nursing model or structure upon which the assessment data were based. Each patient's assessment should be holistic and comprehensive, ie. it should include consideration of the patient's biophysical status, psychosocial status, including cultural, religious and socioeconomic background (where appropriate), environmental factors, self-care and performance of activities of living (what the patient cannot achieve and has concerns about), education and knowledge level of health and present condition.

2. That the nurse's assessment of the patient is a continuous process. Often patients are assessed on the first visit or admission to hospital, but little information is added at a later date. In some situations it may be advisable to set target dates for reassessment, or provide extra space in assessment notes to record additional information.

3. That the patient's problems or concerns about her/his health state are recorded from her/his perspective and the nurse's perspective. Nurses often copy their medical colleagues by only highlighting the patient's main problems according to the medical diagnosis. In addition to recording the patient's own concerns and feelings the nurse should write down what she/he believes the patient's main problems to be.
Nursing diagnostic categorisation has been used to simplify this process, but the nurse should be careful when using this system as it has not yet achieved widespread acceptance in the UK. Doubts have been expressed as to which categories some patient problems fit into and that a system of diagnosing patients' problems is too narrow and rigid.

4. That appropriate nursing care planning has taken place in relation to the interventions necessary to meet the patient's nursing needs. In some situations, eg. day surgery and intensive care, use of 'routine' or 'core' care plans have been devised to

save time recording repetitive, habitual and unchanging nursing activities. These are acceptable as long as individual differences are recorded.

The crucial factor in writing nursing care plans is that they should highlight the proposed nursing actions aimed at helping the patient. They should also contain a unique element which specifies the distinct and possibly exclusive 'personal care' that each individual patient should receive.

5. The progress the patient is making and the sequence of nursing interventions, with appropriate rationale. The patient's progress should be recorded on a regular basis, in a similar way to keeping a diary or log book. These accounts should not be written in a subjective, chatty, or judgemental style. Gossip and hearsay should be avoided; the report should focus on the nurse's observations and relevant patient comments.

    This section of the nursing records is often used in professional and legal wrangles to clarify what has happened and in what order the events took place. Therefore, it is important to not only date and time every written entry but also decide how often to record the information. For example, if there is a sudden change in the patient's condition, ongoing shift recordings will need to be made as well as a summary of events at the end of the shift.

    Nurses working in rehabilitative and long-stay situations should make a daily record of patients' progress. In the community, a summary of each visit should be recorded. This section of the record can be used to record unexpected events, critical incidents and anything that the nurse thinks is relevant to the patient's progress and nursing care.

6. That evaluation of the patient's care has been carried out and reassessed and that the patient has been prepared for transfer or discharge. This is often the most neglected and poorly written section of the nursing records. Evaluation should not be viewed as the final stage of the nursing process. It should be considered as a critical and pivotal activity which sets the scene and standards for continuing the nursing care, and transferring or discharging the patient to another agency.

    All entries relating to evaluation should be clearly labelled, dated and signed. The evaluation should include information based on reassessment by the nursing team, and the patient's/family's/significant others' opinions and observations.

7. That the patient's wishes have been closely followed and respected. The introduction of patient charters and the emphasis on patients' rights and autonomy means that patients' wishes about their treatment and care have to be respected. For example, many patients are now developing written living wills and statements about what should happen to them if they suffer loss of mental capacity or if their condition deteriorates or they are admitted in a 'vegetative' state (see *Chapter 3*).

8. A clear and legible sequence of events. As nursing practice becomes more complex and the need for nurses to document their practice and ideas increases, then the ability to express oneself succinctly in records assumes greater importance. Skill in writing and expression is vital if accurate information is to be correctly interpreted by others (See *Chapters 1* and *2*).

9. The correct date and time of events. All records should be made as soon as possible after a patient has been assessed and evaluated. The practitioner should also sign her/his name after each recording.

In summary, a well-written document will:

(a) Be devoid of abbreviations, meaningless phrases and subjective statements such as 'good day' and 'slept well'

(b) Act as a model for other colleagues' records

(c) Inform all members of the health care team, thus helping in the coordination of interdisciplinary care

(d) Contain direct data from the patient and indirect data from sources such as surgical reports, laboratory tests and consultations

(e) Provide an accurate, evidence-based record of nursing care

(f)   Reflect creativity and individualised patient care

(g)   Evaluate core outcomes and demonstrate modifications
        in nursing plans

(h)   Follow trust and UKCC guidelines.

Auditing nursing documentation

At the start of this chapter, quality assurance was referred to as the method by which performance of nursing care could be evaluated for effectiveness. Performance can be achieved and monitored by nursing audit, peer review and patient satisfaction.

Nursing audit is similar to other forms of health care auditing. It can be either retrospective or concurrent. A retrospective audit is conducted after a patient's discharge or transfer to a new health care situation and involves examining a large number of nursing records. The patient's entire nursing care is evaluated and comparisons made across other cases. Often, a special audit tool is used which asks the reviewer several questions as she/he progresses through the patient's history. Recommendations for change can be made following the analysis of cases and an evaluation of the nursing documentation.

A concurrent audit is conducted during the patient's course of nursing care. It examines the current quality of nursing recording and documentation as well as the care being given to achieve desirable nursing outcomes. Changes can be made if they are indicated and improvements implemented before the patient is discharged.

Figure 4.1 is a simple audit tool which can be used as a rough guide to assessing the quality of nursing recording and documentation. It can help nursing teams to evaluate the current state of their nursing documentation and act as a tool for peer review. Peer review occurs when practising nurses assess performance against standards and criteria that have been previously determined to indicate quality care and documentation. The documentation standards of the UKCC and the key points proposed in this chapter can guide this process.

Patient satisfaction has long been used by institutions to find out how satisfied patients are with the health care services provided. Questions about nursing documentation, the patient's involvement and confidentiality could easily be incorporated into a questionnaire that can be filled out either shortly before or after the patient's discharge.

Summary

The most important aspect of nursing documentation and professional accountability is the setting up of clear standards for practice. The UKCC's guidelines are a helpful start in developing and monitoring local standards but they require local and individual application.

Quality assurance is the method by which performance of nursing care is evaluated for effectiveness. The quality of nursing documentation and reporting can be measured by using appropriate audit forms, peer review and patient satisfaction interview or questionnaires. A significant number of professional conduct cases brought to the UKCC each year cite failure to keep accurate records or report incidents. To ensure good risk management practice nursing documentation standards should be developed and audited appropriately.

Figure 4.1: Castledine Audit for nursing documentation			
Y= Yes; P= Partially; N= No; N/A= Not applicable			
Assessment			
1.	Has a basic nursing assessment of the patient been completed on admission (within 24hours)?	Y P N	
2.	Is there any evidence that the following have been assessed?		
a)	General appearance	Y N	N/A
b)	Hearing difficulties	Y N	N/A
c)	Breathing difficulties	Y N	N/A
d)	Visual difficulties	Y N	N/A
e)	Speech difficulties	Y N	N/A
f)	Circulation	Y N	N/A
g)	Temperature control and vital signs	Y N	N/A
h)	Elimination (bowels)	Y N	N/A
i)	Elimination (bladder)	Y N	N/A
j)	Nutrition	Y N	N/A
k)	Hydration	Y N	N/A
l)	Condition of skin	Y N	N/A
m)	Pressure sore risk assessment	Y N	N/A
n)	Abiltity to wash and dress	Y N	N/A
o)	Problems with mobility/ walking/ moving about	Y N	N/A
p)	Manual handling and lifting rating	Y N	N/A
q)	Prosthesis/aids and appliances	Y N	N/A
r)	Psychological state	Y N	N/A
s)	Social circumstances	Y N	N/A
t)	Perception of illness	Y N	N/A
u)	Family involvement	Y N	N/A
v)	Patient allergies	Y N	N/A
w)	Dressing	Y N	N/A
x)	Rest and sleep pattern	Y N	N/A
y)	Tentative discharge plans	Y N	N/A

Care planning			
3.	Have individualised care plans been written for the patient within 48 hours	Y	N	P
4.	Are the care plans related to the problems identified in the assessment	Y	N	P
5.	Are achievable goals written for the patient?	Y	N	P
6.	Are nursing interventions appropriate and relevant?	Y	N	P
7.	Are nursing interventions in accordance with agreed standards of care?	Y	N	P
8.	Are there evaluation dates?	Y	N	P
9.	Has the care been evaluated when it should have been	Y	N	P
10.	Does the evaluation reflect the patient's progress?	Y	N	P
11.	Evidence of patient involvement	Y	N	P
12.	Evidence carer invlovement	Y	N	P
13.	Is there evidence od a discharge plan?	Y	N	P
14.	Is there evidence of ongoing assessment	Y	N	P

General documentation points			
Diary, daily shift entries of patients' progress. Are they:			
Dated	Y	N	P
Timed	Y	N	N/A
Signed (full sidnature)	Y	N	
Clearly expressed	Y	N	P
Well written	Y	N	P
Black/dark ink used	Y	N	
Entries consecutive and chronological	Y	N	
Meaningless, offensive or subjective phrases used	Y	N	
Good overall picture of the patient	Y	N	
Abbreviations used	Y	N	
Alterations made appropriately, eg. not Tippex	Y	N	

UKCC's *Standards for Records and Record Keeping*

Introduction

1. The important activity of making and keeping records is an essential and integral part of care and not a distraction from its provision. There is, however, substantial evidence to indicate that inadequate and inappropriate record keeping concerning the care of patients and clients neglects their interests through:

   1.1 impairing continuity of care;

   1.2 introducing discontinuity of communication between staff;

1.3 creating the risk of medication or other treatment being duplicated or omitted;

1.4 failing to focus attention on early signs of deviation from the norm and

1.5 failing to place on record significant observations and conclusions.

2. For these reasons the Council has prepared this standards paper to assist its practitioners to fulfil the expectations it has of them and to serve more effectively the interests of their patients and clients.

3. To meet the standards set out in this document is to honour, in this aspect of practice, the Council's expectation (set out in the *Code of Professional Conduct for the Nurse, Midwife and Health Visitor*) that:

As a registered nurse, midwife or health visitor you are personally accountable for your practice and, in the exercise of your professional accountability, must:

1. act always in such a manner as to promote and safeguard the interests and well-being of patients and clients;

2. ensure that no action or omission on your part, or within your sphere of responsibility, is detrimental to the interests, condition or safety of patients and clients.'

The purpose of records

4 The purpose of records created and maintained by registered nurses, midwives and health visitors is to:

4.1 provide accurate, current, comprehensive and concise information concerning the condition and care of the patient or client and associated observations;

4.2 provide a record of any problems that arise and the action taken in response to them;

4.3 provide evidence of care required, intervention by professional practitioners and patient or client responses;

4.4 include a record of any factors (physical, psychological or social) that appear to affect the patient or client;

4.5 record the chronology of events and the reasons for any decisions made;

4.6 support standard setting, quality assessment and audit and

4.7 provide a baseline record against which improvement or deterioration may be judged.

The importance of records

5 Effective record keeping by nurses, midwives and health visitors is a means of:

5.1 communicating with others and describing what has been observed or done;

5.2 identifying the discrete role played by nurses, midwives and health visitors in care;

5.3 organising communication and the dissemination of information among the members of the team providing care for a patient or client;

5.4 demonstrating the chronology of events, the factors observed and the response to care and treatment and

5.5 demonstrating the properly considered clinical decisions relating to patient care.

Standards for records — key features

6 In addition to fulfilling the purposes set out in paragraph 4, properly made and maintained records will:

6.1 be made as soon as possible after the events to which they relate;

6.2 identify factors which jeopardise standards or place the patient or client at risk;

6.3 provide evidence of the need, in specific cases, for practitioners with special knowledge and skills;

6.4 aid patient or client involvement in their own care;

6.5 provide 'protection' for staff against any future complaint which may be made and

6.6 be written, wherever possible, in terms which the patient or client will be able to understand.

Standards for records — ethical aspects

7 A correctly made record honours the ethical concepts on which good practice is based and demonstrates the basis of the professional and clinical decisions made.

8 A basic tenet of records and record keeping is that those who make, access and use the records understand the ethical concept of professional practice which relate to them. These will include, in particular, the need to protect confidentiality, to ensure true consent and to assist patients and clients to make informed decisions.

9 The originator will ensure that the entry in a record that she or he makes is totally accurate and based on respect for truth and integrity.

Standards for records — recording decisions on resuscitation

10 It is essential that the records on the subject of resuscitation accurately and explicitly reflect any wishes of a patient expressed when legally and mentally competent or those of the patient's next of kin or other significant persons when those circumstances do not apply. This is particularly important when

a patient has expressed a wish not to be resuscitated. This is to say that the wishes of a patient, made and expressed when she or he was legally and mentally competent, should be respected.

11 Where the views of the patient and/or those of 'significant others' in relationship to them have not been recorded, but a decision not to resuscitate has been made on clinical grounds by the relevant medical staff, this also should be entered in writing in the medical record and the entry must be signed and dated by the responsible registered medical practitioner. Wherever possible this should be a team decision which, though made by the medical staff, would take the informed views of the nursing staff (and, where applicable, midwifery staff) into account. The patient's family or other significant personal carers should, wherever possible, be consulted.

12 Whether the circumstances in paragraph 10 or paragraph 11 apply, the entry must be able to be located easily and quickly in the medical record and must include a time limit for which it is to apply before review. Nursing and midwifery staff must not enter this decision in the nursing or midwifery record unless it has first been entered in the medical record in the way described in paragraph 11 above.

Standards for records — essential elements

13 In order to fulfil the purpose stated in paragraph 4, to be effective and to meet the standards set out above, records must:

13.1 be written legibly and indelibly;

13.2 be clear and unambiguous;

13.3 be accurate in each entry as to date and time;

13.4 ensure that alterations are made by scoring out with a single line followed by the initalled, dated and timed correct entry;

13.5 ensure that additions to existing entries are individually dated, timed and signed;

13.6 not include abbreviations, meaningless phrases and offensive subjective statements unrelated to the patient's care and associated observations;

13.7 not allow the use of initials for major entries and, where their use is allowed for other entries, ensure that local arrangements for identifying initials and signatures exist and

13.8 not include entries made in pencil or blue ink, the former carrying the risk of erasure and the latter (where photocopying is required) of poor quality reproduction.

14 In summary, the record:

14.1 is directed primarily to serving the interests and care of the patient or client to whom the record relates and enabling the provision of care, the prevention of disease and the promotion of health and

14.2 will demonstrate the chronology of events and all significant consultations, assessments, observations, decisions, interventions and outcomes.

15 In hospitals or other institutions providing care, a local index record of signatures should be held. Where initials are regarded as acceptable for any purpose, these also should feature in the index, together with the full name in printed form.

The 'process' approach or 'planned individualised care' approach to nursing and midwifery care

16 Given the nature of care plans and records associated with the planned individual care approach, this important aspect of records must satisfy the criteria specified in paragraphs 4 to 15 above. The 'process' approach assists a systematic approach to practice. It also provides a framework for the documentation of that practice. The term therefore describes the continuum of distinctly separate yet interrelatd activities of practice, assessment, planning, implementation and evaluation of care.

17 Meticulous and timely documentation provides evidence of the practitioner's actions, the patient's or client's response to those actions and the plans and goals which direct the care of the patient or client.

18 The preparation and completion of care plans will, therefore, in addition to satisfying the criteria set out in paragraphs 4 to 15 above, demonstrate that each step in what is a continuing process has been followed and provides the basis for further goal setting and actions.

19 The making of entries will be organised so that:

19.1 a measurable, up to date, description of the condition of the patient or client and the care delivered can be easily communicated to others and

19.2 the plan and other records complement each other.

20 The practitioner, in applying the process and using the plan, will distinguish between those matters which must be recorded in advance (such as planning and goals) and those which can only be current or slightly retrospective (such as observations and evaluation). Equally, the distinction must be made between entries on papers, (for example, planning forms) which may not be locally retained, and other forms which are part of the clinical nursing or midwifery care records which record changes and events and must be retained.

The legal status of records and its implications

21 Any document which records any aspect of the care of a patient or client can be required as evidence before a court of law or before the Preliminary Proceedings Committee or Professional Conduct Committee of the Council (the UKCC) or other similar regulatory bodies for the health care professions including the General Medical Council, the comparable body to the UKCC for the medical profession.

22 For this, in addition to their primary purpose of serving the interests of the patient or client, the records should provide:

22.1 a comprehensive picture of care delivered, associated outcomes and other relevant information;

22.2 pertinent information about the condition of the patient or client at any given time and the measures taken to respond to identified needs; .

22.3 evidence that the practitioner's common law duty of care has been understood and honoured and

22.4 a record of the arrangements made for continuity of a patient's care on discharge from hospital.

23 Particular care will be exercised and frequent record entries made where patients or clients present complex problems, show deviation from the norm, require more intensive care than normal, are confused and disorientated or in other ways give cause for concern.

24 In situations where the condition of the patient or client is apparently unchanging, local agreement will be necessary in respect of the maximum time allowed to elapse between entries in patient or client records and the nature of those entries. All exceptional events, however, must be recorded and the Council will expect nurses, midwives and health visitors to exercise suitable judgement about entries in the record.

25 Ownership of the contents of a record would normally be seen as residing with the originator of any particular entry. In practice, however, where the professional practitioner is a salaried employee of the health services, the question of ownership turns on ownership of the document on which the record is made. Ownership does not rest with the patient or client, as the creation of law to grant patient or client access in certain circumstances clearly reveals.

26 Midwives must ensure that they are aware of and comply with the requirements in respect of records set out in the Council's 'Midwives Rules'.

27 It is essential that members of the professions must be involved in local discussions to determine policies concerning the retention or disposal of all or any part of records which they or their colleagues make. Such policies must be determined with recognition of any aspects of law affecting the duration of retention and make explicit the period for which specific categories of records are to be retained. Any documents which form part of the chronological clinical care record should be retained.

Retention of obstetric records

28 All essential obstetric records (such as those recording the care of a mother and baby during pregnancy, labour and the puerperium, including all test results, prescription forms and records of medicines administered) must be retained. Decisions concerning those records which are to be regarded as essential must not be made at local level without involving senior medical practitioners concerned with the provision of maternity and neonatal services and a senior practising midwife.

29 Those involved in determining policy at local level must ensure that the records retained are comprehensive (in that they include both hospital, community midwifery records and those held by mothers during pregnancy and the puerperium) and are such as to facilitate any investigations required as a result of action brought under the Congenital Disabilities (Civil Liabilities) Act 1976 or any other litigation.

Patient or client held records

30 The Council is in favour of patients and clients being given custody of their own health care records in circumstances where it is appropriate. Patient or client held records help to emphasise and make clear the practitioner's responsibility to the patient or client by sharing any information held or assessments made and illustrate the involvement of the patient or client in their own care.

31 Evidence from those places where this has become the practice indicates that there are no substantial drawbacks and

considerable ethical benefits to be derived from patients or clients having custody of their records. This immediately disposes of any difficulties concerning access and reinforces the discipline that should apply to making entries in records.

32　A small number of instances will inevitably arise, where a system of patient or client held records is in operation, in which the health professional concerned will feel that her or his particular concerns or anxieties (for example about the possibility of child abuse) require that a supplementary record be created and held by the practitioner. To make and keep such a record can, in appropriate circumstances, be regarded as good practice. It should be the exception rather than the norm, however, and should not extend to keeping full duplicate records unless in the most unusual circumstances.

Patient or client access to records

33　With effect from 1 November 1991, patients and clients have had the right of access to manual records about themselves made from that date as a result of the Access to Health Records Act 1990 coming into effect. This has brought such records into line with computer held records which have been required to be accessible to patients since the Data Protection Act 1984 became operative.

34　These Acts give the right of access, but the health professional most directly concerned (which, in certain cases will be the nurse, midwife or health visitor) is permitted to withhold information which she or he believes might cause serious harm to the physical or mental health of the patient or client or which would identify a third party. The system for dealing with applications for access is explained in the 'Guide to the Access to Health Records Act 1990', published by the Government Health Departments.

35　The Council fully supports the principle of open access to records contained in these Acts, and the guidance notes concerning their operation, and trusts that access will not be unreasonably denied or limited.

36   All practitioners who create records or make entries in any records must be aware of the rights of the patient or client in this regard, give careful consideration to the language and terminology employed and recognise the positive advantages of greater trust and confidence of patients and clients in the professions that can result from this development.

Shared records

37   The Council recognises the advantages of 'shared' records in which all health professionals involved in the care and treatment of an individual make entries in a single record and in accordance with a broadly agreed local protocol. These are seen as particularly valuable in midwifery practice. The Council supports this practice where circumstances lend themselves to it and where relevant preparatory work has been undertaken. Each practitioner's contribution to such records should be seen as of equal importance. This reflects the collaborative and cooperative working within the health care team on which emphasis is laid by the Council in its *Code of Professional Conduct for the Nurse, Midwife and Health Visitor.* The same right of access to records by the patient or client exists where a system of shared records is in use. It is essential, therefore, that local agreement is reached to identify the lead professional to be responsible for considering requests from patients and clients for access in particular circumstances.

Computer held records

38   The application of computer technology should not be allowed to breach the important principle of confidentiality. To say this is not to oppose the use of computer held records, whether specific to one profession or shared between professions. Practitioners must satisfy themselves about the security of the system used and ascertain which categories of staff have access to the records to which they are expected to contribute important, personal and confidential information.

39   Where computer technology is employed it must provide a means of maintaining or enhancing service to patients or clients

and avoid the risk of inadvertent breaches of confidentiality. It must not impose a limit on the amount of text a practitioner may enter if the consequence is that it impedes the compilation of a sufficiently comprehensive record. The case for it has to be considered in association with the questions of access, patient or client held records, shared records and audit. Local protocols must include means of authenticating an entry in the absence of a written signature and must indicate clearly the identity of the originator of that entry.

The practitioner's accountability for entries made by others

40 Irrespective of the type of record or the form or medium employed to create and access it, the registered nurse, midwife or health visitor must recognise her or his personal accountability for entries to records made by students or others under their supervision.

Summary of the principles underpinning records and record keeping

41 The following principles must apply:

41.1 the record is directed primarily to serving the interests of the patient or client to whom it relates and enabling the provision of care, the prevention of disease and the promotion of health;

41.2 the record demonstrates the accurate chronology of events and all significant consultations, assessments, observations, decisions, interventions and outcomes;

41.3 the record and the activity of record keeping is an integral and essential part of care and not a distraction from its provision;

41.4 the record is clear and unambiguous;

41.5 the record contains entries recording facts and observations written at the time of, or soon after, the events described;

41.6 the record provides a safe and effective means of communication between members of the health care team and supports continuity of care;

41.7 the record demonstrates that the practitioner's duty of care has been fulfilled;

41.8 the systems for record keeping exclude unauthorised access and breaches of confidentiality and

41.9 the record is constructed and completed in such a manner as to facilitate the monitoring of standards, audit, quality assurance and the investigation of complaints.

This document is to be revised in 1998/1999

5

Documentation and the nursing process

The origins and development of the nursing process in the UK

Before the introduction of the nursing process in the UK some 20 years ago, nursing practice was poorly recorded and reported (Lelean, 1973). This was often because the scientific and theoretical framework of nursing was weak. Nursing was viewed as a series of functional tasks, many of which were related to medical interventions. Florence Nightingale, in discussing the nature of nursing, observed that 'nursing has been limited to signify little more than the administration of medicines and the application of poultices' (Nightingale, 1859).

The rise of nurse theorists in North America and, in particular, the development of nursing education in universities in the UK has caused a dramatic increase in efforts to define what nursing is and to discover a unique body of professional knowledge.

It is debatable which should have come first: the nursing process or a definition of nursing. McFarlane and Castledine (1982), however, argue that in a society where 'nursing is part of a health care system within a welfare state, it is a complex human activity which defies a simple definition'. Because of this complexity, the nursing process has been accepted as an effective and integral part of the conceptual framework of nursing practice.

In essence, the nursing process is simple and straightforward. 'It combines the most desirable elements of the art of nursing with the most relevant elements of systems theory, using the scientific method' (Shore, 1988). It incorporates problem-solving and decision-making into an interactive/ interpersonal approach (Peplau, 1952; King, 1971; Travelbee, 1971; Yura and Walsh, 1988). The view that the nursing process is a mechanistic or 'staged' approach to determining a patient's problems and planning care is unfortunate. This may have been true in the past and may still be the case in some care situations today. Certainly, when the nursing process was first introduced some nurses saw it as little more than a recording system or a new way of writing. In fact, the nursing process is a dynamic system that can be used to explore the more intricate aspects of individual patients, their holistic needs and the unique outcomes of their health care.

The nursing process was first introduced in North America in the 1950s as a three-step process of assessment, planning, and evaluation based on the scientific method of observing, measuring, gathering data and analysing findings. It was McFarlane (McFarlane and Castledine, 1982) and the 'Manchester nursing movement' who first encouraged its use in the UK in the late 1970s.

Since that time it has undergone years of study, implementation, research and refinement and can be viewed as the interaction between key enabling terms (such as assessment, problem identification, planning, implementation and evaluation) and the care concepts of nursing practice (person, health, environment and nursing).

Nurses should be continually assessing their patients and planning and evaluating care. Although we view the terms assessment, problem identification, planning, implementation and evaluation as separate progressive steps, in reality they are interrelated. This is because nurses are continually with their patients and therefore each stage merges so that the whole process forms a continuous circle or cycle of events.

The model shown in *Figure 5.1* illustrates that the nursing process is an interactive and dynamic action which is constantly changing depending on the individual patient's health, environment and management needs.

Assessment, planning, implementation and evaluation should not be carried out as rigid, systematic and step-by-step stages. In some situations, eg. an emergency, the nurse may have to use all the core elements within a matter of minutes, whereas at other times it may be necessary to dwell on one particular elements, eg. the implementation of one particular nursing intervention.

Figure 5.1: The dynamic and interactive aspects of the nursing process

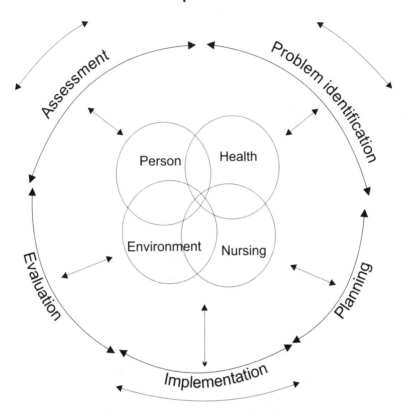

When the nursing process became accepted in British nursing it was generally seen as a four-step process of assessment, planning, implementation and evaluation. Nowadays, it is better to divide the assessment stage into two:

1. The nurse collects data from a variety of sources, eg. other members of the health care team and the patient's family and friends, and carries out physical examination, psychosocial and spiritual assessments.

2. The nurse analyses all the available information, in order to decide, with the patient, the key problems and needs. This is a

crucial stage because it results in a comparison being made between the nurse's perception of the patient's problems and needs and the patient's perception of her/his problems and needs.

To use the nursing process effectively, the nurse must possess and apply important key competences and skills. These include:

◆ Good interpersonal skills and communication with patients

◆ The ability to perform technical skills such as physical and psychosocial assessments based on sound evidential models and tools

◆ A thorough knowledge of science and theory as applied to not only nursing but also other disciplines such as medicine, sociology and psychology

◆ The ability to adapt and be flexible, dynamic and creative when handling patients and their information

◆ The ability to cluster data according to a nursing model and to possess written skills that express and communicate the contribution nursing is making to the patient's general health care state.

The nurse's initial and ongoing assessments should be documented in the patient's record or database. The identification of patient problems/needs, and the planning of patient care, should be recorded in a section of the patient's care plan. The implementation of the plans of nursing, the nurse's observations and patient responses should be charted in progress notes and/or flow sheets. Finally, evaluations of nursing care should be contained in the progress notes or another suitable section. According to Doenges *et al* (1995):

The goals of the documentation system are to:

◆ *Facilitate the delivery of quality patient care*

◆ *Ensure documentation of progress with regard to patient-focused outcomes*

◆ *Facilitate interdisciplinary consistency and the communication of treatment goals and progress.*

For the purposes of communicating and documenting nursing, the core elements of the nursing process help to classify and clarify what has happened or is happening to the patient and what the nursing contribution has been. The nursing process therefore is applicable to a whole range of nursing situations and nursing models and is a way of communicating nursing to the patient and other members of the health care team.

Documenting assessments by nurses

Initial assessment data are usually recorded on special assessment forms. These are generally printed with blank spaces for specific data collection and serve as checklists. In some settings, assessments are written as narrative on blank sheets of paper.

The priority of data collection and assessments is determined by the patient's immediate condition or needs. This is best illustrated in casualty where the triage system is used. Triage was first introduced as a system for dealing with casualties during World War 1 in France. Essentially, triage follows the primary rule of ABC + H, ie. airway, breathing, circulation and haemorrhage. The nurse assessing patients either at the scene of an accident or on admission to casualty must decide which patients require immediate emergency treatment and care. In triage systems practised in hospitals priority is given to those most critically injured. However, because of the sheer numbers involved in mass casualty triage, priority is given to the most seriously injured who have the best chance of survival (Judd and Ponsell, 1982).

The writing up of a triage assessment or report is just as important as the documentation of any other nursing assessment. It should include: the patient's response; the nature of the presenting situation; care rendered; and anecdotal notes. Its function is to provide information which can help answer questions at a later stage. In most cases the written assessment follows key headings or questions which are provided on special forms developed by the emergency care directorate.

Pertinent data should be collected using appropriate assessment techniques and the nurse qualified accordingly. Data collection and assessment should involve the patient, significant others, and health care providers when appropriate. The whole process must be systematic and ongoing, although it is important to establish baseline data.

The initial database must be designed according to the environment in which it is used and the type of patient nursed. For example, if most patients admitted to a medical/surgical unit are elderly, the database should focus on the common problems seen in this patient population, such as being at high risk of skin breakdown, falls and sensory impairments.

In the community, nurses have to be sensitive to local environmental variations, housing and social needs. The time-frame for completing the initial assessment is defined by local policy and varies according to the needs of the patient population and clinical area. For example, emergency patients are usually assessed immediately, whereas an individual who is being admitted for long-term therapy may be assessed over a period of hours or even days.

Priority assessment issues

As a result of the increasing demands made on hospital beds and the trend towards shortened lengths of stay in hospitals there is now, more than ever before, a need for efficient and adequate collection of data and assessment. Iyer and Camp (1995) suggest that nurse assessors should focus on the four priority 'Ps' of assessment:

1. Problems: the patient's priorities

2. Patient's risk of injury

3. Potential for self-care following discharge

4. Patient and family education needs.

The principle of nursing reassessment or ongoing assessment is dependent upon the potential for change in the patient's/client's health care state. However, even in long-stay situations, all patients should be regularly reviewed. *Table 5.1* outlines patient types and the suggested times for carrying out a reassessment of their condition.

Table 5.1: Suggested times for reassessment of patients	
Type of patient	**When to reassess**
Stable medical/surgical patient	As required
Acute medical/surgical patient	Ongoing
Long-term care patient	As required
Rehabilitation patient	Every 1 to 2 weeks, depending on progress
Same-day surgery patient	On return from theatre and immediately before discharge, depending on condition
Patient with decreasing neurological status or acute accident victim	Every 15 minutes, or when required
Suicidal patient	Continuously on a one-to-one basis
Patient with gastrointestinal bleeding	Continuously

Adapted from Springhouse Corporation (1995)

Documenting planning

Written records take on special significance because they are used as the basis for giving care and serve as a communication tool for everyone involved in patient care.

The style of care plans varies within each care situation. Most plans use a column format. The titles of these columns have changed over the years to reflect trends in nursing language. The first major column is usually labelled 'Patient problems or nursing diagnosis'. The second major column has changed from 'Nursing goals' to 'Patient outcomes'. The third column may be labelled 'Plan of care', 'Nursing action', 'Nursing orders' or 'Nursing interventions'. These latter terms are interchangeable but 'Nursing interventions' is presently recommended. Therefore we now have:

Patient problems/ Nursing diagnosis	Patient outcomes	Nursing interventions

Additional columns may be added to the care plan for date, signature, outcomes achieved and date care plan was changed or revised. Some care plans have columns for evaluation comments whereas others rely on the progress notes for such appraisal. With the increasing use of computers in health care, many institutions have computerised care plans.

Standard care plans for commonly occurring problems are in common use. However, these should not be a substitute for individualised nursing care and therefore a separate or additional space may be needed for recording patients' individual needs.

Narrative report writing in progress notes is the traditional and accepted method of recording what has happened to a patient. The order of recording is generally the order in which events occurred. For example:

> *7/4/96, 1300 hours: Tried to get out of bed with one nurse, however, this required assistance of two people. Patient complained of feeling very dizzy when sitting on edge of the bed. Observations of vital signs were stable and after a couple of minutes patient able to stand with assistance. Walked several steps with the help of two nurses. Sat out in chair for 10 minutes and then helped back into bed by one nurse. Dressing to abdominal wound changed. Incision site dry, clean and no sign of infection or problems. S Beatles, Staff Nurse.*

The relevance of nursing diagnosis

The definition of nursing diagnosis is not universally agreed and its application to nursing in the UK has not been accepted. Its use arises from the American Nurses' Association's (ANA's) definition of nursing:

Nursing is the diagnosis and treatment of human responses to actual or potential health problems (ANA, 1980).

The North American Nursing Diagnostic Association (NANDA) approved the following definition of nursing diagnosis in March 1990:

A nursing diagnosis is a clinical judgement about individual, family, or community responses to actual or potential health problems/life processes. Nursing diagnosis provided the basis for selection of nursing interventions to achieve outcomes for which the nurse is accountable (Carroll-Johnson, 1990).

The key words are critical thinking, clinical judgement and decision-making. The following are some examples of approved NANDA diagnoses: high risk of infection; constipation; diarrhoea; stress incontinence; urinary retention; high risk of injury; high risk of impaired skin integrity; social isolation; sexual dysfunction; high risk of caregiver role strain; spiritual distress; impaired physical mobility; fatigue; feeding self-care deficit; body image disturbance; pain; chronic pain; anxiety; and fear. All of these can be used as the basis for planning nursing interventions. Whether or not they are used, it is important that the patient's problems are stated clearly, concisely and accurately.

In the UK, the use of the term 'diagnosis' is generally accepted as the identification of disease by means of a patient's symptoms. The association of this term with medicine and the fear of wrongly labelling patients, has caused some British nurses to be sceptical about its use. Perhaps it is preferable to refer to nursing diagnosis as 'problem identification'. Having made this point, however, it is important to recognise that one of the major difficulties for nurses in the UK is stating and writing down the patient's nursing problems.

Many nurses confuse medical diagnosis with the identification of the patient's nursing problems. For example, the main focus for nursing problem identification is monitoring how the patient is responding to actual or potential health problems; the focus of the medical and collaborative health care teams, however, is on monitoring the pathophysiological and medical response of the body organs or system *(Table 5.2)*.

Table 5.2: Differences between nursing and medical roles		
	Primarily the nursing role	**Primarily collaborative and medical role**
1. Focus of assessment activities	Focus on monitoring patient's nursing response to actual or potential health problems and concerns	Focus on monitoring pathophysiological and medical diagnostic response to medical treatment and medical problems
2. Problem identification	To identify and confirm that a problem or concern exists that is solely the responsibility of the nurse	To identify and confirm the medical diagnosis. Some nurses may be qualified or trained to assist in this process, but the final decision belongs to the physician

3. Treatment and care	The nurse decides the most appropriate nursing intervention and care based on sound nursing evidence and research	The physician decides on the most appro- priate medical intervention and the nurse collaborates to give medical treatment and care
4. Accountability	The nurse is accountable for all nursing treatment and care	The doctor is accountable for all medical treatment and care

Three comparisions of the nursing problem identification with collaborative problems and medical diagnoses are now given with an exercise on identying nursing, collaborative and medical problems.

Nursing problem identification

Nursing problem identification involves either using the principles of the nursing diagnosis system or focusing on the nurturing, caring and holistic aspects of the patient's needs and responses to health/illness.

Medical problem identification (ie. medical diagnosis)

Medical diagnosis is the formal statement or labelling of the identification of a disease or mental condition, that is validated by medical diagnostic studies and for which the treatment is determined by a registered medical practitioner, eg. a fracture, chronic bronchitis and depression.

Collaborative health problem identification (ie. the concern of the whole health care team)

Collaborative health problem identification is the recognition by one member or all members of the health care team that an actual or potential health care problem exists which is the responsibility of the whole team. The team may decide that one particular individual or profession should take responsibility for dealing with the problem, eg. the patient's reaction to her/his medical diagnosis.

Exercise

Identifying nursing problems, collaborative problems and medical diagnosis

For the following statements write at the end of the problem if you think it is primarily a nursing problem (NP), collaborative problem (CP), or medical diagnosis (MD).

1. Potential problem of pressure sores due to bony prominences
2. Potential problem of bleeding now the patient is on anticoagulant therapy
3. Increased intracranial pressure due to secondary concussion
4. Pneumothorax
5. Difficulty expectorating sputum
6. Difficulty coping with grief responses
7. Loss of interest/involvement in activities of self-care
8. Lacks appropriate stimulation/cognitive experiences
9. Chest infection
10. Unexplained/progressive weight loss
11. Unsafe gas/electrical appliances
12. Pain in operation site
13. High risk of falls
14. Failure to adapt to lifestyle as a result of a health problem
15. Anxiety and fear related to separation from parents
16. Alzheimer's disease
17. Depression due to loss
18. Potential problem of low pulse due to digoxin therapy
19. Difficulty in taking an adequate intake of fluid by mouth

20. Knows how to empty drainage bag but not how to irrigate the catheter

Answers

1: NP	2:CP	3:CP	4:MD	5:NP
6:NP/CP	7:NP	8:NP	9:MD/CP	10:CP
11:CP	12:NP/CP	13:CP	14:CP	15:NP/CP
16:MD	17:MD	18:CP	19:NP	20:NP

Key points when identifying nursing problems

◆ Do not let interdisciplinary or multiprofessional problems compromise unidentified nursing problems

◆ Interdisciplinary or multiprofessional problems require collaboration with other health care professionals (eg. physician, surgeon, physiotherapist, dietician, occupational therapist, speech therapist, social worker, clergy)

◆ Depending on the setting and the patient population, there may be more or fewer interdisciplinary problems than there are nursing problems

◆ The relationship between nursing problems and interdisciplinary problems is not always easy to separate.

Evidence-based care planning

The plan of nursing care should guide care as well as document the planning phase of the nursing process. Evidence-based care planning is an approach to decision-making in which the nurse uses the best evidence available, in consultation with the patient, to decide upon the option which is most suitable for the patient.

Scientific and practice principles provide the rationale for nursing interventions. Current research findings and carefully thought through nursing interventions, in collaboration with the patient where possible, enable the best evidence-based care to be put into practice. Practice guidelines or nursing protocols should be based on the best evidence available as these are often used to guide specific nursing interventions.

In the past, nursing care was generally based on custom and practice or opinions dominated by values and resources. Today, and into the next century, nurses will have to practice evidence-based decision-making because patient expectations are rising and the demand for high quality health care is expanding.

The general purpose of evidence-based nursing is to select from the health-related literature articles which demonstrate that there is a need for change in nursing interventions. This critical appraisal of the literature is the rationale for change in practice and should always be done in consultation with professional colleagues and involve the patient if possible. Recording the use of research in practice will strengthen and support the nurse's situation if ever she/he is called upon to answer questions about her/his professional nursing care.

Methods of keeping records

There are various ways in which nursing information can be recorded. The key difference between them is the manner in which the information is organised. Apart from using their own records, nurses may also contribute to medical and multidisciplinary documentation. Although these are institutional records, it is important to remember that anything written or printed may be used as evidence in a court of law.

Whatever system or method is used, the following nursing information should always be available:

1. Admission or first contact/visit, nursing history.

2. Collection of data about the patient/client relating to physical state, psychological/emotional condition and relevant spiritual and social history.

3. Nursing problem identification and professional nursing judgements.

4. Nursing care plans.

5. Diary-style progress record of nursing care, therapy, treatment, observations and evaluations.

6. Evidence that the nurse has tried to involve the patient and her/his significant family or friends, if appropriate.

7. Ongoing use of the principles behind the nursing process and, where relevant, information relating to transfer and discharge.

Problem-orientated medical records (POMR)

This method of documentation was originally developed by Dr Lawrence Weed in North America in 1969. It places the emphasis on the patient's/client's problems and the required interventions. Originally, the POMR model was intended for physicians, but later it was adapted for use by all members of the health care team and was referred to as the problem-orientated record (POR).

The components of POR include:

1. A database about the patient/client

2. A problem list

3. An initial plan

4. Progress notes, written in SOAP format (ie. subjective, objective, assessment, plan).

Each member of the health care team contributes to a single list of identified patient/client problems. There is a common, coordinated plan of care and all team members complete the progress notes.

SOAP Notes

S = subjective data

What the patient/client verbally expresses to the nurse

O = objective data

What the nurse observes about the patient's/client's behaviour, clinical condition, etc.

A = assessment

The conclusion or nursing judgement reached regarding a patient's/client's condition based on both the subjective and objective data

P = plan

The nurse's plans for the patient/client which have been reached by agreement with the patient/client.

Following modifications, the letters IER have been added to the basic SOAP approach.

I = intervention

This indicates a particular action by a discipline

E = evaluation

This reflects the patient's/client's response to her/his health care problems/concerns and nursing interventions

R = revision

Changes to the original plan of care that are made as necessary.

Therefore, the system can be written as SOAPIER. The advantages of the SOAPIER system of progress writing are that:

(a) It can be adapted to fit rapidly changing patient situations

(b) It reflects the elements of the nursing process

(c) It focuses on the patient/client and her/his problem

(d) It encourages efficiency in gathering data about patients/clients from all caregivers

(e) It makes it easier to follow a patient's/client's progress because the problem are listed and labelled with numbers

(f) It encourages patient/client involvement in her/his care and problem identification

(g) It encourages greater continuity of care among the multidisciplinary health care team

(h) It demands continuous evaluation and revision of the care plan.

One of its major disadvantages is that the whole health care team needs to be trained in the system. Unfortunately, some nurses become lazy when using this system, leaving the bulk of the writing and comments to other members of the team.

Focus charting

Focus charting is another method of recording nursing information, which was also developed in North America by Susan Lampe (1994). This approach emphasises the use of a focus column which includes any topic, words or phrases from the nurse's assessment of the patient's/client's situation. The column helps the user to organise information quickly and may include concerns other than just the patient's/client's problem (see *Figure 5.2*).

According to Lampe (1994), there are four essential elements in focus charting:

◆ *Focus*: identifies the content or purpose of the narrative entry and is separated from the body of the notes in order to promote easy data retrieval and communication

◆ *Data:* the subjective and/or objective information supporting the stated focus or or the description of the observations at the time of a significant event

◆ *Action*: describes the interventions past, present and future of the health care team member

◆ *Response*: describes the patient outcome/response to interventions or describes how the care plan goals have been obtained.

The words or phrases used in the focus column can vary, but usually they relate to the patient's response and not her/his medical diagnosis.

Figure 5.2: Example of focus charting system		
Column for:		
Date/time	**Focus**	**Patient progress notes**
10.01.96	Incisional plan	Data: patient complains of abdominal pain of 7 on scale of 10
10.00		Action: pethidine 100mg given
11.00		Response: resting in bed. States pain has decreased to a rating of 3

Other examples of information which can be included in the focus column are:

Admission to hospital ward
Return from surgery
Discharge planning
Shortness of breath
Medication teaching
Anxiety about health condition
Self-care deficit in feeding
Angry outburst
Confusion in time, place and person
Emotional support
Potential complication of paralytic ileus
Atrial fibrillation

As a result of the wide variety of charting methods in patient care, there is a danger that information will become fragmented. For example, often the nurse has to look at several different forms in order to gather all the information she/he needs to nurse the patient. Focus charting is one answer to this problem because it provides a summary of the overall condition of patients/clients and their progress towards a certain goal or outcome. It also helps the nurse to think in terms of the nursing process, which means that care is based on the patient's needs. Focus charting is flexible enough to be used in all settings, including critical care and home nursing.

The use of the word 'focus' instead of 'problem' creates greater flexibility; the focus could be on anything from a patient behaviour to a concern, need, task, incident or event. Another advantage of this method is that categories of data, action and response are not required for each focus cited, and therefore charting is made much easier.

The disadvantage of this system, as in most structured progress note systems, is that some nurses have difficulty in documenting information and distinguishing which data should be placed in the appropriate columns.

Other methods of record keeping

There are other methods of record keeping in existence, but these are not as structured as the SOAPIER and focus systems. All, however, contain sections which broadly follow the nursing process and contain a mixture of medical, social and nursing information.

The most important element of all systems is the progress notes. This regular diary of events was lost in the transition from the former Kardex system to the nursing process of care. Confusion existed in relation to when to evaluate care plans, how often, and where to include data relating to ongoing events and patients' progress.

Progress notes

The increase in complaints and legal actions has made it advisable to maintain regular progress notes. These should include all significant events that occur, during either the patient's hospitalisation or transfer home while she/he is receiving nursing care and medical treatment. The notes should be written clearly and objectively and reflect the patient's progress towards desired measurable outcomes. Furthermore, they should:

◆ Describe incidents and events and emergency situations

◆ Describe patients' behaviour and responses to nursing care and treatment

◆ Contain direct quotations from patients/clients and their significant others as is deemed appropriate by the nurse

◆ Follow on from each other without breaks or gaps, describing the progress that the patient/client is making

◆ Not contain meaningless subjective phrases such as 'Good day' and 'Satisfactory'.

From the notes, the reader should be able to form a clear picture of what has occurred to the patient. The best way to ensure the clarity of progress notes is through the use of descriptive (or observational) statements.

Examples of judgemental language

She/he is paranoid when we go into her/his room.

Remains uncooperative today.

Very confused.

Addicted to analgesics.

She/he is a manipulative patient.

Has a poor outlook on life.

Depressed and unwilling to cooperate.

Good night.

Examples of objective statements

Donald expresses anger to the nurses by shouting and swearing at them.

Mary is uncooperative because she refuses to let the nurse help her with her identified problems.

Bill is confused in time, place and person according to the assessment tool.

Jane is demanding more analgesia than she has been prescribed.

David tries to goad the rest of the patients into supporting his view.

Derek is very concerned about the effect of his diagnosis on his future lifestyle.

Ann is sad, and says she feels like dying.

Tom says his pain is like a red hot poker.

Mary says she did not sleep at all last night.

Remember, whatever you write in the progress notes will have an impact upon future care. Future carers will have to rely on your written words if they are to share your understanding of the patient's situation at a given moment (Doenges *et al*, 1995).

Content of successful progress notes

The progress notes must contain any information that is of importance to oncoming shifts as well as observations that the nurse has made which may be of significance to other health care providers. The following are examples by Doenges *et al* (1995) of the kind of information that should be included:

◆ *Unsettled or unclear problems or 'issues'* that need to be dealt with, including attempts to contact other health care providers

◆ *Noteworthy incidents or interviews* involving the patient that would benefit from a more detailed recording

◆ *Other pertinent data* such as notes on telephone conversations, home visits and family interactions

◆ *Additional critical incident data* such as seemingly significant or revealing statements made by the patient, insights into a patient's patterns of behaviour, patient injuries, the use of any special treatment procedure, or other major events such as episodes of pain, respiratory distress, panic attacks, medication reactions or suicidal comments

◆ *Administered cure activities or observations* if not recorded elsewhere on flow sheets (physician visits, completion of ordered tests, non-routine medications, etc).

Remember the importance of correct grammar and spelling, legible entries, using black, indelible ink and writing the patient's name on each chart. Finally, remember that entries need to be concise and precise, ie. use succinct sentences or phrases that provide enough information to communicate your observations, thoughts and judgements.

Evaluation

Progress notes should contain an evaluation of patient outcomes. There are two types of evaluation: formative and summative. As outlined in *Chapter 1*, formative evaluation occurs during the provision of nursing care and is carried out on an ongoing basis, whereas summative evaluation occurs at the end of an activity, eg. following discharge or transfer or at the conclusion of a particular phase of nursing, such as intensive therapy or rehabilitation.

The frequency of formative evaluations depends on the condition of the patient and the expected timeframe of changes in the patient's condition. The number, type and intensity of nursing interventions is another guide as to how often the nurse should be writing progress notes. Obviously, the greater the number and variation the more frequent the evaluation.

Summative evaluations include the degree to which the patient was involved in her/his care and the patient's response to health education and teaching. Discharge or transfer summaries should include the instructions, treatments, nursing care activities, medications and follow-up appointments that the patient has been given by the nurse. These days there is increasing support for patients signing that they have received this information and understood what the nurse has said to them.

Key points when reporting and recording information

1. Information should be accurate, concise, organised, pertinent, current and complete.

2. Language should be direct, simple and geared to the level of the receiver.

3. Focus should be on the interchange and understanding of the information exchanged.

4. Personal attitudes or judgemental language should not enter into professional communication.

5. Non-professional, obscure or inflammatory terms should be avoided.

6. Information should be presented in chronological order and contain formative and summative evaluations.

High-risk patients

Patients who are at risk of injuring themselves or others are a concern for all nursing staff. It is important when assessing a patient or taking a nursing history that the nurse listens carefully for any particular clues and records potential problem areas. In children this may be signs of child abuse, physical problems, poor home safety, or bad behaviour.

Older adults may suffer physiological changes in vision, hearing, mobility and circulation which may predispose them to falls and other accidents. In addition, they may also be at risk of elder abuse and ageism. Confused or disorientated patients demand special consideration; the use of physical restraints such as special belts or ties is not encouraged in the UK. However, if a patient is unconscious and at risk of falling out of bed or from a stretcher, then the use of side rails is advised (Holden and Woods, 1982).

Difficult and high-risk patients should be assessed not only at home or on admission, but also periodically throughout their stay in hospital or long-term care facility. When recording information about high-risk patients it is important to note why they have been put in such a category.

Patient assessments should include:

(a) The reasons why special nursing observations are needed

(b) The use of any particular nursing control, method, device or restraint

(c) Whether the patient is receiving any medication that is controlling her/his behaviour, or which may affect her/ his balance, mobility or alertness

(d) The type and method of restraint used

(e) The patient's response, outcome or safety and the continued need for restraint.

Falls

It is important that all health care personnel are alerted if a patient is at increased risk of falling. In some organisations, ribbons, stickers, or notices are used to identify such patients. With regard to documentation, the nurse should ensure that the risk is recorded in a prominent place in the patient's assessment and care plan.

Risk assessments should be recorded routinely on vulnerable patients and should include:

◆ Level of consciousness

◆ Orientation to time, place and person

◆ Balance

◆ Mobility

◆ Precautions taken to prevent falls — by assistance or restraints

◆ The use of medications which may increase the likelihood of falls

◆ Relevant observations by staff and family members.

In all cases where nurses are dealing with patients who are at risk of injuring themselves or others, it is essential that they not only use their clinical judgement and assessment skills, but also write down their decisions based on the potential for injury assessment and risk management.

Discharge and transfer of high-risk patients/clients

The following are categories of patients/clients who are particularly at risk when being transferred between health and nursing services. It is therefore important to make sure that information about the individual is adequately documented.

1. Patients/clients who lack knowledge about their own medical and nursing treatment/care plans.

2. Patients/clients newly diagnosed with a chronic disease.

3. Patients who have undergone major/radical surgery.

4. Patients in need of prolonged recuperation and convalescence

5. Patients at risk of social isolation and lack of support.

6. Patients with a history of emotional or mental instability.

7. Patients requiring a complex home care regimen.

8. Patients from diverse ethnic and cultural backgrounds.

Discharge summaries

It is important that the nurse who has been responsible for a particular patient completes the patient's discharge summary. She/he should focus on the resolution of the nursing problems and how well the patient achieved the desired nursing outcomes. This will complement the information contained in the doctor's discharge letter which usually emphasises the course of the patient's illness and the medical treatment prescribed.

Discharge instruction sheets are used in a variety of settings; it is important that these include a written record of what was said to the patient on discharge. Malpractice suits have been initiated as a result of poor discharge information being given to patients and their family/significant others. Therefore, the nurse must record carefully what she/he has said, document if the patient refuses to listen to instructions, and signs that follow-up health/nursing information has been given.

Key points

1. Nursing is concerned with wholeness and health in humans. It recognises that people are continuously interacting with their environment.

2. Problem identification and professional nursing judgement are vital components of the nursing process. The stages of the nursing process are:

    i)   Collection of data

    ii) Assessment of data

    iii) Problem identification and professional judgement

    iv) Planning

    v)   Implementation

    vi) Evaluation.

3. Problem identification is linked to the professional judgement of the nurse. It is this link that is the key to deciding what are nursing, collaborative and medical problems.

4. The process of professional judgement involves diagnostic reasoning and includes the activities of:

    i)   Collecting information

    ii) Clustering information

    iii) Writing down clearly appropriate statements about these clusters.

5. Conceptual frameworks, nursing models, lists and statements about the properties of nursing help provide a focus for the

process of stating and writing down clearly those activities for which the nurse is responsible.

6. An acceptable definition of nursing diagnosis which includes professional judgement and problem identification is as follows:

   A nursing diagnosis is a clinical judgement about an individual, family, or community that is derived through the process of nursing and provides the basis for the type of care, therapy, or treatment, for which nurses are accountable (adapted from Shoemaker, 1984).

7. Nursing judgements should always be clearly expressed, and documented in nursing records and collaborative care records.

6

Computer charting, community documentation and conclusions

Computer charting

In health care, the emphasis is now on developing computerised clinical nursing record systems. Although the principles laid out in this book deal primarily with written documentation they can be easily transferred to computerised systems. Computerised documentation is an ideal way of dealing with large volumes of patient information.

The best way to learn about computerised systems is to get hands-on experience. The advantages are:

♦ Enhanced data management and communication

♦ Reduced clerical work

♦ Greater organisation and work efficiency

♦ Reduction in medication errors

♦ Enhanced teaching of patient care management

♦ Enhanced development of protocols by checking and updating evidence-based information

♦ Legibility

♦ Accuracy

♦ Rapid interdepartmental communication and improved communication with general practitioners in community clinics

♦ Reduced errors.

The disadvantages are:

◆ Malfunction

◆ Dehumanisation or the impersonal effects of having to deal with a machine all the time

◆ Concern for confidentiality and privacy. the problem of security and access is the subject of much discussion in the uk

◆ Cost of the system

◆ Computer lag during peak usage and an inadequate number of terminals

◆ Nurses may be reluctant to give up written notes.

With traditional record keeping, access to information is restricted simply by keeping the record in the unit or clinic. With a computerised system of record keeping such information can be retrieved by anyone who has the ability to seek entry into the system or through 'hacking', ie. the act of breaking into a computerised system. Examples of the methods being developed to stop unauthorised entry include: complex passwords or computer signatures; special timing devices that shut down a terminal; special back-up files; and reminding users to keep the time they leave information about a patient displayed on a monitor to a minimum.

Despite all these efforts, more people have access to computerised records than have access to handwritten records. This is of great concern and as nurses we must be aware of these dangers and the laws and rules of confidentiality.

Key rules for computer documentation

The use of computers means that the pen has been replaced with an electronic entry system (keyboard, light pen, touch pad, mouse) and printer. The date and time may be recorded automatically or may need to be typed in.

The nurse's signature is often coded into the computer. Alternatively, the nurse may have a personal access code. Never share your computer signature or code and never chart under someone else's code. All entries should be legible and accompanied by a date, time and signature code. When mistakes are made or you feel that you have typed in the wrong information, record 'error' or 'correction' to the dated entry and add your alteration or reassessment. *Do not* record unsupported value judgements or inferences or obliterate or try to erase errors in computer systems which are programmed to prevent unauthorised entries.

When computers are introduced into clinical situations it is important that the whole nursing team is trained and educated in their use.

The future

It is difficult to predict the ways in which nursing documentation will change as a result of computerisation. Standardised medical protocols or treatment orders may be built into computer records. This means that a nurse could initiate treatment and care as soon as a patient arrives in hospital, or is seen in the home environment. Developments in software may result in nurses putting patients into standardised routes of nursing care, with core plans already available on screen. Voice–activated computerised medical records hold great promise for faster documentation of patient care in busy settings. Finally, there is the possibility of computer networks linking up to every home in the country.

The demand for good electronic documentation systems is growing rapidly. However, it is essential that nurses improve their basic documentation skills first.

Community nursing care documentation

Although much of this book has used examples from the hospital environment the fundamental principles of writing and documentation apply equally to the community nursing situation. However, certain factors are specific to nursing in the community.

The nursing process system is more individualised in the patient's home because of the very nature of how nursing is delivered. First, the nurse is a guest in the patient's/client's home and nursing care is not witness by anyone else except those rendering the care, the patient and perhaps the patient's/client's family. Therefore, the only way other people can know what has taken place is by reading the nursing records. If the nursing records are poor, incomplete or inaccurate then a distorted picture of the patient's condition and nursing care will result. Comprehensive documentation is therefore essential for continuity and quality monitoring of nursing in the community.

When a large number of health and social care professionals are involved in caring for a patient and her/his family in their own home then a multidisciplinary care plan must be used which is left with the patient/client. The type of information contained in community nursing records is similar to that in hospital documentation and is influenced by the UKCC's standards, scope of nursing practice, local requirements and clinical condition of the patient/client. In addition, there should be information relating to the reason for the referral and the nursing input.

A detailed assessment should be made of not only the patient/client but also the home environment, safety measures, types of community services, supplies and equipment needs. If relevant, the attitude of the caregiver and/or the family should be included as should the contact person in the case of difficulties or emergency other items to note should include:

- ◆ Directions to the home, access to the premises and entry to be used by the nurse

- ◆ The position of the patient's bed and toilet facilities

- ◆ The need to make any physical adaptation to the accommodation such as a ramp or widening doorways for wheelchair use

- ◆ Pets in the home, including type, number and where housed, eg. outside in a kennel

- ◆ Environmetnal characteristics including size of rooms, assessment of cleanliness, food availability and safety hazards, eg. throw rugs, clutter, dangerous open fires and electric and gas appliances

♦ Support systems, eg. local pub or club or church involvement

♦ Names, addresses and numbers of friends and neighbours who can help if necessary.

Leaving the patient's care plan in the home is very helpful. However, some nurses dictate their visits or record them more fully when they have left the care situation. The longer the period of writing up following the visit, the more likely the possibility of inaccuracies or incompleteness. The use of the SOAP system of record keeping (see *Chapter 5*) is a helpful way for multidisciplinary health care teams to function, as this system can be left in the home and involves the patient's family. Portable computers may be helpful in the future but there is the danger that these may not link up well or be lost or stolen.

Continuing care documentation

Continuing care remains an ambiguous concept both in its definition in professional and policy literature and in its operationalization in practice (UKCC, 1997).

Continuing care usually refers to long-care or chronic disease management. The principles of documentation in this sphere of practice are identical to many of the principles outlined for community nurses both in this chapter and the rest of the book. Progress notes are still the primary means of communication between nurses and other members of the health care team. Whether the long-term care of patients/clients is in their own home or in a nursing home, it is important that their progress is monitored and evaluated. This can be done by frequent summative evaluations and reassessments of the nursing conditions to determine whether there is a need for change in nursing input. Usually, this proccess should be carried out every 3–6 months or depending on a change in the clinical status of the patient. All clinical nursing records and aspects of the nursing process should be updated at intervals based on the seriousness of the patient's/client's condition and be in accordance with recommendations and standards set by authorities such as the local nursing home inspectorate and the UKCC.

Conclusions

This text can be used by all nurses in either the classroom or the clinical situation. It has drawn together some of the most important aspects of writing and documentation for nurses. In particular, it has emphasised the importance of 'nursing' and of identifying nursing's unique contribution to health care.

Multidisciplinary care planning and shared patient records are only as good as the individuals who write them. Sometimes nurses tend to stand back and let the more dominant members of the health care team take charge of the written input into documentation. However, it is essential that nurses make a significant contribution to documenting health care in order to emphasise the nurse's perception of the patient's/client's situation. Nurses' basic competencies and skills in writing will improve only if they practise their skills under the supervision of a more experienced practitioner.

The importance of good interpersonal skills when developing documentation knowledge is emphasised in *Chapter 2*. It is essential to listen carefully to what patients, their family and significant others are saying. Often nurses hinder or inadvertently obstruct good communication because they are in too much of a hurry to do other things. Avoiding professional jargon and clarifying what the patient/client has said are key points.

Changing shift patterns in hospitals means that there is often not enough time for adequate handover and report sessions. This book has emphasised the importance of developing the skills necessary to cope with these changes and of focusing on the most relevant and essential data.

Verbal communication does have certain drawbacks. It does not always allow participants to prepare visually, reflect, organise their thoughts or check that the information is complete before the verbal exchange is finished. In order to communicate well verbally and give efficent reports nurses must consider what they want to say, why, where, when and how they are going to say it. During a report it is always crucial to know when to speak and when to listen.

The key point in relation to effective reporting of information is the importance of making people feel comfortable and committed to listening. Presenting data both verbally and in writing at the participant's level of understanding is essential to the successful imparting of information. Details about patients should be personalised and all data treated with respect and confidentiality.

Discharge and transfer of information between health care agencies is critical for high quality patient care. In the past, filling in the relevant form was viewed as the main medium for transferring vital information. This book has tried to get away from the idea that there are ideal forms and formats for documenting patient/client information. The nurse is encouraged to think carefully and to consider key criteria which can guide more comprehensive record keeping and the exchange of information.

There is no absolute way of doing things, only key principles to be considered. This is particularly the case when writing letters and/or accounts of patients'/clients' progress.

Legal and ethical considerations have been outlined in a simple and pertinent manner. For example, the ethical flower grid (see *Chapter 3*) should help practitioners to reflect on some of the key issues. Unfortunately, in today's health care world, nurses have to spend a great deal of time writing and documention nursing care. Veracity and confidentiality are two ethical principles which apply directly to the documentation of patient information. Nurses have a duty to tell the truth in their reports and an obligation to keep all patient information confidential. In the event of a law suit, the nursing record may form the basis for the plantiff's case, the nurse's defence or the health care organisation's response. Many solicitors now believe that the nursing progress notes are the most fruitful source of proof that significant events occurred. A strong record can be an effective defence for the nurse accused of malpractice or professional misconduct.

The inclusion of the UKCC's *Standard for Records and Record Keeping* (see *Chapter 4*) provides the reader with a comprehensive approach to documentation standards.

In the UK, the nursing process approach has been in existence for over 20 years. At one time it was seen as being too rigid and theoretical and just a paper exercise. However, the core principles are as relevant today as they have ever been. Assessment by nurses has improved to the extent that many nurses have the potential to become experts in physical examinations and psychosocial skills. The nursing process is a dynamic and interactive system which can be used flexibly by nurses on a continuous basis. Patient assessment is a critical part of nursing and identifying the patient's potential and actual nursing problems is crucial to quality health care.

Methods of record keeping and, in particular, the various approaches to recording a patient's progress are reviewed in *Chapter 5*. It is important for nurses to experiment with methods such as 'problem-orientated records' and 'focus charting'. Patients and their families will continue to be at risk and suffer from poor nursing care if the principles outlined in this book are not acted upon and implemented in the UK over the next few years.

Task forces for documenting change

To initiate changes in a nursing documentation system and to regularly monitor and update the process, a task force can be set up. This should comprise representatives from each clinical nursing speciality, nursing management, staff development, education and practitioners. Staff nurses have more realistic perspectives on documentation whereas managers and educators have greater insight into legal and professional conduct issues and strategies for implementation and education.

The purpose of a local documentation task force is to explore the current documentation system, identifying its strengths and weaknesses and to gather data and develop strategies. Using audit tools the group can compare its findings with those of other organisations who have evaluated their systems. The findings can also be compared to standards set by national bodies such as the UKCC. A task force has the potential to reduce duplication, improve quality, standardise forms and reduce charting times and health care risks.

Key points

1. A properly documented health/nursing record should describe all aspects of care that have been carried out for the patient.

2. Correct documentation should:

    i)   Provide evidence that continuity of nursing care began on admission or on the first visit and continued thereafter. the nursing process should be used in a systematic way to avoid haphazard assessment, planning and recording.

    ii) Provide evidence to others (eg. members of health care teams, patients' relatives, solicitors, quality assurers, and the UKCC) that care was carried out carefully and systematically.

    iii) Provide written rationale for the care and treatment recieved and record the patient's responses.

    iv) Provide ample evidence for peer review, clinical supervision, audit and evaluation of nursing..

    v)   Use the best evidence available and the latest research findings

    vi) Provide a legal and professional record that could be used to protect the patient, the organisation or trust, or any members of the health care team (remember, the UKCC may use nursing records as evidence in a professional misconduct hearing).

3. The following is a sequence of statements that the nurse should consider when reflecting on her/his nursing care and the link with writing and documentation:

    i)   Assess patients' problems by interviewing, observing and examining/inspecting

    ii) Ensure that patient assessment is an ongoing process in which you continually review the patient's problems

    iii) Try to involve the patient and her/his significant others whenever possible

    iv) Emphasise the value of 'nursing' throughout your documentation

v)   When you have collected information about a patient identify her/his nursing problems (sometimes referred to as a nursing diagnosis)

vi)   Avoid labelling, medicalising or standardising patients' problems according to narrow categories such as disease processes. Think holistically and treat patients as individuals

vii) Always evaluate your patient's progress. Use progress notes to record how the patient feels about her/his care and treatment. Do not be afraid to change your approaches if they are not working

viii) Always document your patient care assessments and findings as soon as possible

ix)   Always show that you are accountable for your assessments by signing your name on the notes you have completed

x)   Always quote the patient or family member directly if you fear that paraphrasing the information they have imparted will make it lose some of its meaning

xi)   Always write or print legibly, in indelible ink

xii) Always be precise and concise

xiii) Never use abbreviations that may be confused with ones that have an alternative meaning

xiv) Think of your documentation as a camera that takes the patient's picture. Be so specific that anyone who reads your notes will be able to see the patient through your words

xv)   Do not use vague terms such as 'good', 'normal', 'adequate', 'improving', 'better', 'worse' or 'sufficient'

xvi) Always review each of your patient's problems in the progress notes.

xvii)   Ask yourself:

What have I heard?

What have I seen?

What do I think?

What will I do?

What have I done?

How did the patient respond?

xviii) Never let long periods elapse without charting information otherwise it may look as if the patient was neglected during that time

xix)   Never insert notes between lines or leave an empty space for someone else to insert information

xx)   Never change written records to cover up for your own or someone else's mistakes.

The primary purpose of the nursing record is to ensure continuity of quality care to the patient. It must communicate needed information for quality multidisciplinary health care.

7

References and recommended reading

Access to Medical Reports Act (1988) HMSO, London

Access to Health Records Act (1990) HMSO, London

ANA (1980) *Nursing: A Social Policy.* ANA, Kansas City

BMA (1993) *Medical Ethics Today: Its Practice and Philosophy.* BMA, London

BMA (1995) *Advance Statements about Medical Treatment.* BMJ, London

Bolam *vs* Friern Hospital Management Committee [1957] 2 All ER 118 (1957) 1 WLR 582

Carroll-Johnson RM (1990) *Classification of Nursing Diagnosis: Proceedings of the Ninth Conference.* JB Lippincott, Philadelphia

Castledine G (1986) A stress adaptation model. In: Kershaw B, Salvage J, eds. *Models for Nursing.* John Wiley & Sons, Chichester: 55–68

Castledine G (1994) A definition of nursing based on nurturing. *Br J Nurs* **3**(3): 134–5

Creighton H (1986) *Law Every Nurse Should Know.* Saunders, Philadelphia: 54–285

Data Protection Act (1984) HMSO, London

Department of Health (1991) *The Patient's Charter.* HMSO, London

Department of Health (1995) *The Patient's Charter.* HMSO, London

Diers D (1994) What is Nursing. In: McClosky JC, Grace HK eds. *Current Issues in Nursing.* Mosby, St Louis: 5–14

Doenges ME, Moorhouse MF, Burley JT (1995) *Application of Nursing Process and Nursing Diagnosis*, 2nd edn. FA Davis Co, Philadelphia

Egan G (1976) *Interpersonal Living: A Skills/Contract Approach to Human-Relations Training in Groups.* Brooks/Cole, Monterey, CA

Fischbach FT (1991) *Documenting Care, Communication, the Nursing Process and Documentation Standards.* Davis, Philadelphia

Fletcher JA, Gowing DF (1987) *The Business Guide to Effective Writing.* 2nd edn. Kogan Page, London

Gowers E (1956) *The Complete Plain Words.* HMSO, London

Gries A, Currell R (1995) *A Strategy for Security of the Electronic Patient Record,* Version 2.1, Feb Draft. Institute for Health Informatics, Aberystwyth

Henderson V (1966) *The Nature of Nursing: A Definition and its Implications for Practice, Research and Education.* Macmillan, New York

Holden VP, Woods RT (1982) *Reality Orientation.* Churchill Livingstone, Edinburgh

House of Lords (1994) *Report of the Select Committee on Medical Ethics.* HMSO, London

Iyer PW, Camp NHC (1995) *Nursing Documentation: A Nursing Process Approach,* 2nd edn. Mosby, St Louis

Judd RL, Ponsell DD (1982) *The First Responder.* Mosby, St Louis

Keatings M, Smith BO (1995) *Ethical and Legal Issues in Canadian Nursing.* Saunders, Toronto

King IM (1971) *Toward a Theory of Nursing.* John Wiley and Sons, New York

Lampe S (1994) *Focus Charting, 6th edn.* Creative Nursing Management Inc, Minneapolis

Lelean SR (1973) *Ready for Report Nurse.* RCN, London

McFarlane JK, Castledine G (1982) *The Practice of Nursing Using the Nursing Process.* Mosby, St Louis

Meleis AF (1985) *Theoretical Nursing: Development and Progress.* Lippincott, Philadelphia

Molloy W, Mepham V (1993) *Let Me Decide.* Penguin, Harmondsworth

Nightingale F (1859) *Notes on Nursing: What It Is and What It Is Not.* Republished 1946. Lippincott, Philadelphia

NJPC (1979) *Brief Description of a Demonstration Project to Establish Collaboration or Joint Practice in Hospitals.* NJPC, Chicago: 2–6

Peplau HE (1952) *Interpersonal Relations in Nursing.* Putnam, New York

Sereno KK, Bodakin EM (1975) *Understanding Human Communication.* Houghton Mifflin, Boston

Shoemaker JK (1984) Essential features of nursing diagnosis. In: Kim MJ, McFarland GK, McLane AM, eds. *Classification of Nursing Diagnosis, Proceedings of the 5th Conference.* Mosby, St Louis: 104–15

Seedhouse D (1988) *Ethics: The Heart of Health Care.* John Wiley and Sons, New York

Shore LS (1988) *Nursing Diagnosis: What Is It and How To Do It* (a programmed text). Medical College of Virginia Hospitals, Richmond

Springhouse Corporation (1995) *Mastering Documentation.* Springhouse, Pennsylvania

Travelbee J (1971) *Interpersonal Aspects of Nursing,* 2nd edn. F.A.Davis, Philadelphia

United Kingdom Central Council for Nursing, Midwifery and Health Visiting (1992a) *Code of Professional Conduct for the Nurse, Midwife and Health Visitor.* UKCC, London

United Kingdom Central Council for Nursing, Midwifery and Health Visiting (1992b) *The Scope of Professional Practice.* UKCC, London

United Kingdom Central Council for Nursing, Midwifery and Health Visiting (1993) *Standards for Records and Record Keeping.* UKCC, London

United Kingdom Central Council for Nursing, Midwifery and Health Visiting (1996) *Guidelines for Professional Practice.* UKCC, London

United Kingdom Central Council for Nursing, Midwifery and Health Visiting (1997) *The Nursing and Health Visiting Contribution to the Continuing Care of Older People.* UKCC, London

Weed LL (1969) *Medical Records, Medical Education and Patient Care: The Problem-Orientated Record as a Basic Tool.* Case Western Reserve University Press, Cleveland

Yura H, Walsh B (1988) *The Nursing Process.* Appleton-Century-Crofts, New York

Recommended reading

Alfaro R (1990) *Applying Nursing Diagnosis and Nursing Process.* 2nd edn. Lippincott, Philadelphia

Burnard P (1992) *Writing for Health Professionals.* Chapman and Hall, London

Christensen PJ, Kenney JW (1995) *Nursing Process Application of Conceptual Models.* 4th edn. Mosby, St Louis

Clinical Skillbuilders (1992) *Better Documentation.* Springhouse, Pennsylvania

Cormack DFS (1984) *Writing for Nursing and Allied Professions.* Blackwell Scientific, Oxford

Dening J (1986) *Readymade Business Letters.* Kogan Page, London

Edelstein J (1996) A study of nursing documentation. *Nurs Manage* **21**: 40–6

Fletcher J (1983) *How to Write a Report.* Short Run Press, Exeter

Fondiller S (1991) The new look in nursing documentation. *Am J Nurs* **91**: 65–76

Kolin PC, Kolin JL (1980) *Professional Writing for Nurses.* Mosby, St Louis

Marrelli TM (1966) *Nursing Documentation Handbook*, 2nd edn. Mosby, St Louis

Martin KS, Scheet NJ (1992) *The Omaha System: A Pocket Guide for Community Health Nursing.* WBSaunders, Philadelphia

Meyer C (1992) Bedside computer charting. Inching toward tomorrow. *Am J Nurs* **92**: 38–42, 44

NHS Training Directorate Pack (1993) *Just for the Record. A Guide to Record Keeping for Health Care Professionals.* NHS Training Directorate, Bristol

Appendix

A key checklist for charting

1. Ensure the patient's name and identification number are on all health care records

2. Enter the date, time and full signature on all entries including nursing care plans

3. Follow the stages of the nursing process and check that documentation includes the following stages:

   ◆ Assessment

   ◆ Problem identification

   ◆ Planning — nursing care plans

   ◆ Implementation and progress notes

   ◆ Evaluation and audit

   ◆ Reassessment or ongoing assessment information.

4. When writing up assessments include:

   ◆ Initial impressions

   ◆ Head-to-toe physical health

   ◆ Psychological health

   ◆ Sociocultural health

   ◆ Spiritual health

   ◆ Summary of major health concerns and/or problems.

5. Guidelines for judging priorities:

   ◆ First, actual or imminent life-threatening concerns

◆ Second, actual or potential health-threatening concerns.

6. Components of a nursing plan are:

◆ Nursing problem

◆ Expected outcome

◆ Nursing orders

◆ Evaluation.

7. **SOAPIER** system of progress notes:

S — *Subjective data*: client statements and interactions

O — *Objective data:* nurse's observations and measurements

A — *Analysis*: status of nursing problems

P — *Plan of care*: outcome and actions planned

I — *Implementation*: actions implemented

E — *Evaluation*: client responses to action/outcomes

R — *Revision*: changes in plan when necessary.

8. Key things to document:

◆ Activities of living/functional needs

◆ Mental health needs/problems, disabilities

◆ Psychological status/stress adaptation/coping

◆ Pain

◆ Continence

◆ Skin condition and pressure sore risk

◆ Wound status/drainage/appearance

◆ Input and output: fluids and food

◆ Weight and nutrition

◆ Bowel function

- ◆ Vital signs
- ◆ Special treatments
- ◆ Medications/side-effects/allergies
- ◆ Right patient, right medication, right dose, right route, right time
- ◆ Social/environmental needs/problems/protection
- ◆ Spiritual needs
- ◆ Pertinent patient conversations/interviews
- ◆ Pertinent friends/family of the patient — conversations and interviews
- ◆ Significant events — transfer, discharge
- ◆ Changes in condition and status, incidents, unusual and unexpected events
- ◆ Patient education and degree of help needed from nurse — response to teaching, type of information given and patient response
- ◆ Patient — completely independent; requires use of equipment or device; requires help, supervision or teaching from another person; dependent.

9. Always write legibly in indelible ink
10. Do not erase — just cross out if a mistake is made
11. Be precise, concise and specific at all times.

Exercise and study questions

1. What are the key components of nursing documentation?
2. What are the six purposes of documentation?
3. What should nursing progress notes include?
4. List the advantages and disadvantages of computerised documentation.

5. How is nursing documentation related to the nursing process?

6. What is the difference between an initial assessment and an ongoing assessment in nursing?

7. List the areas of assessment to be considered when gathering information for patient discharge or transfer.

8. List the stages of the nursing process that are mentioned in this book.

9. When standardised care plans are used by nurses what should the nurse always consider?

10. List some of the important factors about nursing care plans.

11. Why is it important to make a statement or nursing diagnosis of the patient's problems?

12. What should clinical nursing progress notes reflect?

13. Regardless of the format, what should be included on every nursing record?

14. What should a mental checklist for writing descriptions on clinical progress notes include?

15. What do SOAP, SOAPIER and POMR mean?

16. What are the four essential elements of focus charting?

17. Two of the most common types of litigation are...?

18. What are two of the most frequent problems with nursing charting?

19. Discuss the differences and similarities between law and ethics?

20. Which common characteristics of documentation pose a legal risk?

21. What factors influence the way nurses document?

22. What are two of the key ethical principles that directly relate to reporting?

23. What would you look for in a nursing record if you were the plantiff's expert professional witness in a trial?

24. What are the essential factors you need to know about a patient before commencing nursing care?

Answers

1. *Assessment*
   Nursing problem statement
   Planned care nursing interventions
   Patient teaching, patient outcomes and interdisciplinary communication.

2. *Communication*
   Legal protection
   Professional standards and professional justification for actions to UKCC
   Education
   Quality assurance or quality improvement
   Research.

3. *Patient's condition and complaints*
   Identified problems and concerns
   Nursing interventions and patient response to care
   Diary of the progress the patient is making.

4. Advantages:
   Legibility
   Accuracy
   Timely
   Fast
   Disadvantages:
   Computer malfunction
   Impersonal
   Cost
   Confidentiality concerns.

5. *Shows nursing care is more than a task system*
   Shows each step/stage of the patient's care
   Shows the integration and communication of what nursing is and what is happening to the patient
   Shows the quality and effectiveness of nursing

      Shows holistic nature of nursing
      Shows patient involvement in care.

6. *The first is completed on admission for immediate needs.*
      The latter is built up over time and helps to determine continuing needs.

7. *Patient's medical and nursing condition*
      Ability of the patient to care for self
      Family/friends' support
      Psychosocial status
      Patient's culture
      Future environment of care
      Medication and drugs.

8. *See Chapter 5.*

9. *The patient's individualised needs.*

10. *They should:*
      Be goal directed
      Help in coordination of care
      Help in continuity of care
      State patient's needs
      State nursing intentions or proposed interventions
      Help in shift reporting
      Help in discharge planning
      Help in team conferences.

11. *Lists patient's priorities*
      Identifies nursing concerns and needs
      Clarifies the nurse's thinking and analysis following assessment of the patient's data.

12. *Patient's problems*
      What was assessed
      Clinical data
      Interventions
      Patient responses and outcomes.

13. *Date, time, signature of the nurse.*

14. *Who, what, why, when, where and how.*

15. *See Chapter 5.*

16. *Focus column*
Data
Action
Response.

17. *Negligence, malpractice.*

18. *Omissions, alterations, illegibility and inaccuracies.*

19. *See Chapter 3*
Laws are mandatory
Ethics are guidelines we ought or are obliged to follow.

20. *Illegibility*
Lines or spaces between entries
Improper signing, countersigning or not signing
Tampering
Different handwriting or obliterations
Dates and times of entries omitted
Inconsistent documentation
Use of abbreviations
Subjective and unsupported comments.

21. *The UKCC's standards*
Government regulations/guidelines
Court cases
Trust management
Quality assurance findings.

22. *Veracity*
Confidentiality.

23. *Information relating to patient assessment, reassessment, planning, implementation and evaluation of nursing*
Inadequate documentation
Evidence of negligence and malpractice
Involvement of the patient and significant others
A systematic account or diary of what has occurred
Evidence of patient education and good discharge planning
Nursing actions based on reasonable decisions given the circumstances at the time

Accurate charting of vital signs and key observations relating to the patient's condition

24. *Immediate nursing/medical condition*
   Nursing assessment data and information
   Patient and nursing care priorities
   Evidence–based interventions to meet patient's needs
   Nursing care already provided by other caregivers
   Patient's responses and outcomes of nursing and medical care
   Patient's abilities and degree of involvement.

Test yourself

Mark for √ true and x for false

1. Use white out to completely erase the errors you have made in records ☐

2. Sign, date and time all entries ☐

3. All nursing records can be used in a court of law as legal evidence ☐

4. Events should be recorded chronically and the reasons given for any decisions made ☐

5. Records should be made as soon as possible after the events to which they relate ☐

6. Nursing records should only be written in professional jargon ☐

7. Abbreviations should be used whenever possible ☐

8. The patient/client should be involved whenever possible in the recording and documentation of nursing care ☐

9. Veracity and confidentiality are not ethical principles which apply to nursing documentation ☐

10. Any document which records aspects of patient/client care can be used as evidence in courts of law and at professional conduct committees ☐

11. Patients/clients have the right of access to all nursing records ☐

12. You should document exact quotations from a patient ☐

13. Standardised care plans should be 'rubber stamped' by a nurse and not individualised to the patient ☐

14. A general principle in legal aspects of documentation is: 'If it is not documented, it was not done.' ☐

Answers

1:F	2: T	3: T	4: T	5: T	6: F	7: F

8: T	9: F	10: T	11: T	12: T	13: F	14: T

The Castledine Nursing Model as applied to acute surgical nursing

Physical assessment

State significant characteristics and deviations from norm

Factors	Pre-op assessment	Post-op assessment
1.Overview		
General appearance		
Mobility/movement/posture		
Hands		
Arms		
Shoulders		
Baseline observations		
T P R		
B/P		
Apex rate		
Weight (kg)		
Ward urinalysis		
S.G		
pH		
ALB.		
Sugar		
Acetone		
Blood		
Bilirubin		

Factors	Pre-op assessment	Post-op assessment
2. Head and neck		
Face		
Scalp and neck		
Eyes (pupils)-sight		
Ears-hearing		
Mouth-speech		
(Condition)-teeth		
Nose-smell		
3. Chest		
General shape		
Breathing function		
Heart function		
Breasts (eg.lLumps, prev. mastectomy		
4. Abdomen		
Function (eg. vomiting/ nausea		
Appetite (difficulties)		
Condition of bowel function (eg. distention)		
5. Groin and buttocks		
G.U. function		
Urinary pattern		
Condition of genitalia		
6. Legs		
Muscular function		
Comparitive size		
Walking distance		
impairment		
Condition of skin (colour)		

Factors	Pre-op assessment	Post-op assessment
7. Feet		
Condition of skin		
Nails		
Toes		
8. Skin		
General condition		
Sensory disturbances		

Psychosocial assessment

Factors	Pre-op assessment	Post-op assessment
1. Interpersonal		
1.1 Changing role at home work caused by hospital/illness		
1.2 Level of interdependency A) who shares your (the patient's) feelings, hopes, disappointments? B) Are they available to you now? C) Can we help you in any way? D) Teaching information required?		

Factors	Pre-op assessment	Post-op assessment
2. Intrapersonal 2.1 Feelings about present admission to hospital — including anticipated fears, pleasures		
2.2 Self-concept A) Feelings/experiences related to illness and physical self eg. body image, bodily sensations sexuality, feminity masculinity B) Feelings/experiences related to personal self eg. i) ways illness/surgery has changed the way the patient feels about her/himself ii) what does the patient believe in?(spiritually) iii) what are the patient's expectations following surgery?		
2.3 Pain Painful experiences and sensations		
2.4 Sleep Feelings of tiredness Sleep pattern		
2.5 Stress A) Do you(the patient) understand the term stress? B) What do you find stressful? C) How do you usually cope?		

Overall psychosocial impression of the patient by nursing staff:
(date and signed)

Pre-op:

Post-op:

Examples of documentation

Nursing Process Documentation					
Admission date	Time	Ward	Title/sex	Unit no.	
Surname	1st forename		2nd forename	Marital status	Religion
Home address				Post code	
Tel. number	Next of kin		Relationship	Address/Tel. no.	
Consultant	Speciality		Category of patient	DOB	Age
Surname at birth	Place of birth		Source of admission	Management intention	
Occupation of patient		Date of waiting list		Date resident in UK	
Family doctor		Referred to		Address from which admitted	
Allergies/sensitivities				Valuables Yes/No	
Past medical history/operations					
Current medical diagnosis					
What patient thinks reason is for admission					
Investigations and date		Operations performed and dates			
Discharge plan (home circumstances — support services/medical social worker/physiotherapy/transport/medication/OPD appointment)				Lay carer: Tel. no.	
			Information taken by: Grade: Date & Time: Given by:		

Nursing Process Documentation

Model of care:		Patient's name	Unit no.
NEED/PROBLEM	AIM/OBJECTIVE	PLAN OF CARE	DISCONTINUE

NB. CANCEL PLANS WITH A BOLD RED ‡

Nursing History

SURNAMES: FORENAMES: RECORD No:

LIKES TO BE REFERRED TO AS:

DATE OF ADMISSION TO HOSPITAL: WARDS
                                 WARDS

NEXT OF KIN: RELEVANT Tel. Nos.

DATE OF BIRTH: G.P:

AGE:

MEDICAL DIAGNOSIS:
CONSULTANT:

REASON FOR ADMISSION:

WHAT PATIENT OR FAMILY UNDERSTANDS ABOUT HIS/HER CONDITION:

PATIENTS AND/OR FAMILY REACTIONS TO HOSPITAL ADMISSION:

MEANINGFUL PERSON IN LIFE — SIGNIFICANT OTHERS/PETS:

MEALS ON WHEELS ETC. COMMUNITY RESOURCES (D.N., H.V., SOCIAL WORKER:

RELIGIOUS PRACTICES OR BELIEFS PT. FINDS HELPFUL:

RECREATIONAL ACTIVITIES AND PAST WORK LIFE:

GENERAL HEALTH HISTORY AND PREVIOUS HOSPITAL ADMISSIONS:

GENERAL ASSESSMENT ON ADMISSION

ASSESSMENT FACTORS

		HOSPITAL N0.
DATE	NAME	NURSE

HISTORY OR USUAL CONDITION/BEHAVIOUR

DATE COMMENCED	PATIENT'S NURSING PROBLEM	EXPECTED OUTCOME	NURSING CARE PLAN	DATE DISCONTINUED

NAME   HOSPITAL N0.

NAME		HOSPITAL NO.			
DATE ORDERED	PARA-NURSING INVOLVEMENT & MEDICAL INVESTIGATIONS	DATE COM-PLETED	DATE	PROGRESS/EVALUATION	

Index